D1558814

Genetics and American Society

Kenneth M. Ludmerer

Genetics and American Society
A Historical Appraisal

The **Johns Hopkins University Press**
Baltimore and London

Copyright © 1972 by The Johns Hopkins University Press
All rights reserved. No part of this book may be reproduced or transmitted in any
form or by any means, electronic or mechanical, including photocopying, recording,
xerography, or any information storage and retrieval system, without permission in
writing from the publisher.
Manufactured in the United States of America

The Johns Hopkins University Press, Baltimore, Maryland 21218
The Johns Hopkins University Press Ltd., London

Library of Congress Catalog Card Number 72-4227
International Standard Book Number 0-8018-1357-3

Originally published, 1972
Second printing, 1974

Library of Congress Cataloging in Publication data will be found on the last printed
page of this book.

To My Parents

Contents

Preface

This book is a social history of genetics in the United States. It explores the impact of the science on American society, particularly through the utilization of genetic theories to determine social policy, and the repercussions of social and political events for the study of genetics. It is my hope that this book will help elucidate the manner in which science and society interact generally and provide perspective on political and social issues of the 1970's which involve biological questions.

In preparing this volume, I was concerned principally with attitudes. I wanted to discover how the popularization of theories of heredity influenced the social views of the general public, and how in turn the "genetic" justification of political and social positions affected geneticists. To do this, I turned as much as possible to manuscript material. The personal papers of a number of geneticists, deposited at the American Philosophical Society Library, provided considerable insight into the views of geneticists toward political events involving their science. I derived further understanding from many persons involved with the events discussed in the book. R. A. Brink, Emanuel Celler, F. A. E. Crew, James Crow, C. D. Darlington, L. C. Dunn, Harry Harris, Lancelot Hogben, Walter Landauer, Lionel Penrose, J. A. Fraser Roberts, Curt Stern, and Sewall Wright graciously consented to be interviewed. Others, particularly John Z. Bowers, F. Clarke Fraser, Arno Motulsky, James V. Neel, Clarence P. Oliver, Frederick Osborn, Sheldon C. Reed, Herschel L. Roman, William J. Schull, Laurence H. Snyder, Carl J. Witkop, and Stanley W. Wright, were kind enough to correspond with me over the matter.

In writing this book I have profited from the generous assistance and encouragement of many individuals. Lloyd G. Stevenson made the volume possible by appointing me a Fellow in the Institute of the History of Medicine of the Johns Hopkins University so that I might pursue the project without interruption. He was a continual source of insight and understanding, and he offered useful criticisms of all drafts of the manuscript. Everett Mendelsohn introduced me to the study of the relationships of science and society and provided much assistance throughout my investigations. Conversations with Mark Adams, Gert Brieger, Barton Childs, Yehuda Elkana, Jerome Frank, Judith Grabiner, Victor McKusick, and Herbert Odum also stimulated many ideas presented in this book. Professors Childs and McKusick commented on the written manuscript as well. Saul Benison, Donald Fleming, Sheldon C. Reed, and James R. Schaber offered detailed and helpful criticisms of the entire book; Lancelot Hogben and Lionel Penrose made suggestions for those portions relating to human genetics. Janet Koudelka patiently answered my innumerable questions on style, and Robert Zelenka carefully read the entire work for consistency and form. Eula Bartlebaugh expertly did the typing. To these and many other persons I am grateful.

This project was supported by P.H.S. Training Grants 5 T01 LM 00105-10 and 2 T01 LM 00105-11 and by a Henry Strong Denison Award from the Johns Hopkins University School of Medicine. A grant from the National Genetics Foundation enabled travel to England related to the book.

Abbreviations

The following abbreviations have been used in the footnotes:

CBD: Charles B. Davenport Papers
American Philosophical Society Library

LCD: Leslie C. Dunn Papers
American Philosophical Society Library

HSJ: Herbert S. Jennings Papers
American Philosophical Society Library

EAR: Edward A. Ross Papers
State Historical Society of Wisconsin

IRL: Files of the Immigration Restriction League
Box I, Houghton Library
Harvard University

Correspondence: Correspondence of the House Committee on
Immigration and Naturalization
68th Congress
National Archives

Genetics and American Society

1

Introduction

Perhaps no science in modern times has had so great a social impact and has been so enmeshed in diverse social issues as genetics. Ideas of heredity have influenced psychology, sociology, history, education, and literature as well as the religious and social attitudes of the general public. Currently, genetic theories applied to agriculture have produced the "green revolution" with its potential to save millions from starvation; in the past, misapplied genetic theories culminated in the Nazi extermination of millions of people. Because the laws of genetics are valid for human beings as well as other organisms, the science of genetics itself has been vulnerable to social and political intervention. At no time has a more dramatic interference with the science occurred than in the late 1940's and 1950's, when the Soviet government for political reasons sanctioned Trofim Lysenko's erroneous genetic theories and censured those who disagreed.

I propose to examine a central and significant interaction of genetics and society: the use of genetic theories as a justification for various laws, and the consequences of political events for the development of genetic science. The focus is primarily upon the United States, where the main episodes have occurred, though parallels and contrasts are drawn with events elsewhere. I hope that this analysis will contribute to a greater understanding not only of the relationship between genetics and society but of a major theme in American social history as well. In assuming a prominent role in the justification of the Immigration Restriction Act of 1924, genetic theories helped end a policy of immigration fundamentally important to the nation's growth and development. The debates over immigration restriction are important not only in their own right as a major landmark in American social history, but also as part of a larger tradition of conflict in United States history between the country's democratic ideals of liberty, equality, and opportunity for all and the reality of repres-

1

sion for some. This conflict has manifested itself in different ways: morally, in the long-continuing displacement and suppression of the Indians; economically, in slavery and selective immigration restriction; politically, in the Alien and Sedition Acts of 1798 and of World War I. Other events are so complex that no single category suffices: the deportation of alleged radicals following World War I, the deposition of Japanese-Americans in concentration camps during the World War II, and the McCarthy phenomenon of the fifties.

* * *

To understand the social history of genetics, it is necessary to discuss the eugenics movement. In America the movement began shortly after 1900, being an outgrowth of the naturalistic climate of the late nineteenth century. Historically, the term "eugenics" has meant many things: a science which investigates ways to improve the genetic condition of the human race; a program to promote such improvement; a social movement; and a pseudo-scientific sanctuary for bigots and racists. When used in an unqualified context in this book, the term "eugenics" refers strictly to the American social movement of that name, which enjoyed greatest influence between approximately 1905 and 1930 and which advanced a two-part program of "negative eugenics" (preventing the reproduction of those regarded as "unfit") and "positive eugenics" (encouraging the reproduction of those considered "fit") to promote racial betterment. Concern about man's genetic future was not confined to this period, but only then did the problem have enough popular appeal to sustain a politically influential movement.

In this book three major themes are developed. First, what were the circumstances, both scientific and social, which between 1905 and 1930 drove many Americans to look to the science of genetics as a guide for legislation? Since most of the leading proponents of biologically based legislation belonged to the eugenics movement, it is important to understand in detail the motivations, aspirations, and attitudes of the eugenicists as well as the degree to which their legislative suggestions were valid in terms of the genetic knowledge of the day. The attitudes of geneticists and human geneticists of the era toward the eugenics movement are also of importance here.

Second, how were genetic theories utilized, primarily by eugenicists, to gain support for the passage of various laws? Between 1905 and the early 1930's eugenic arguments were advanced for a variety of types of legislation ranging from prohibition to birth control. Here three pieces of legislation were particularly important because on no other issue was there so much agreement among the eugenicists and on no other issue was the biological justification so articulately advanced. These were the eugenic sterilization laws (which by 1931 had been passed in thirty states), the Immigration Restriction Act of 1924 (also called the Johnson Act), and the eugenic sterilization law of Nazi Germany. Strictly speaking, the "biological justification" of these laws misrepresented genetic science, but the public widely believed it. I do not attempt to ascribe to "genetic" theory a pre-eminent role in the passage of those laws; the biological justification was one of several important factors behind them, and I am aiming to understand just what purpose it served. Proponents of those bills entertained many motives in addition to the biological one; nevertheless, genetic theories played an essential role. I hope that this discussion will help elucidate an important general question, the use of science as an instrument of social policy.

Finally, there were three principal situations in which social and political events affected the activities of geneticists in America. Two of these events occurred in the late 1920's and 1930's, involving eugenicists' use of "genetics" as a justification of social programs of dubious scientific and ethical value. First, eugenicists' misuse of genetic science became so blatant that many prominent geneticists felt obligated to step outside the laboratory and denounce the movement publicly. In so doing some of these geneticists became the first group of scientists anywhere to raise the question of what constitutes the investigator's social responsibility concerning the social applications of his discipline. Second, at the same time in the late 1920's and 1930's, eugenicists' misuse of genetic science had the additional effect of inhibiting research in the area of human genetics. From the start eugenicists had dominated the field of human genetics; as the movement fell into disrepute, the reputation of human genetics for a while fell along with it. After World War II, social events influenced genetics a third time when the advent of the atomic age greatly stimulated the growth of human genetic studies. Throughout the 1940's the field of human genetics had been steadily progressing of its own accord, but after the war it benefited enormously from the vast amount of attention it received from a public alarmed over the genetic hazards of radiation for mankind.

In pointing to the repercussions of these social circumstances on the science of genetics, I have not assumed a social determinist stance. The progress of a science cannot be explained completely in terms of the social demands placed upon it, though instances in the history of science can indeed be found where the desire to meet pressing social needs underlay important scientific discoveries.[1] My general intention here is to discover ways in which social and political events can influence the course of a science. Though discussion of internal laboratory developments is fundamental to writing the history of a science, too often are external social factors overlooked.

Much of this book discusses ideas of various persons on the subject of race. At the turn of the century anthropologists commonly defined a human race as a group with common physical and anthropometric characteristics. Most workers at this time tended to exaggerate the extent and significance of racial differences. They divided mankind into a large number of racial types, including three races of Europeans which will be met later in the book; and they postulated that all races are descended from hypothetical ancient "pure types" and that differences among the races are large and unalterably fixed by heredity. A great number of them believed that races possess characteristic mental as well as physical qualities and that certain races are innately "superior." Beginning around the mid-1920's, many anthropologists, prompted by Franz Boas and his students, began to re-examine such views on race. Though they continued to define a race in terms of its physical characteristics, they also recognized that the differences between races are small compared to the similarities, that there is more variation within a race than between races, and that the many intermediate grades of variation between races make the distinction between them an arbitrary one. They further realized that an individual is a product of his environment and upbringing as well as his "innate biological nature." These latter views are essentially correct, though since 1940 they have been extensively revised by the application of genetics to the study of human races. Today a human race is best defined not in physical but in genetic terms—namely, as a population which differs significantly from other human populations in regard to the frequency of one or more of the genes it possesses. With the aid of genetic tools, especially the analysis of blood groups, anthropologists now divide mankind into six main genetic races (Early European, Caucasian, Negroid, Mongoloid, American, and Australian), having achieved a much greater theoretical understanding of the nature of racial differences and similarities.[2] This

1. Among these instances are the development of thermodynamics from the technological problems of the German cannon industry and Pasteur's discovery of fermentation while assisting the French wine industry.

2. The definition of race given here is taken from William C. Boyd, *Genetics and the Races of Man* (Boston: Little, Brown and Co., 1953), p. 207. To classify all Caucasians as one race is not to say that there are no subgroups within the race, merely that the differences among the subgroups are too slight to justify their each being labeled a separate race.

reorientation in the study of human races is but one part of a general restructuring within anthropology which has resulted from the application of genetic analysis.[3]

In many places in the book it will be important to determine whether particular individuals were "racists." Without a precise definition of the word, this undertaking would be impossible. The main difficulty with the term is that its usage has changed with time. Discussion of racial superiority and inferiority in mid-nineteenth century America can be understood adequately only in the context of a theological debate; this early racism differed in nature from the literary and nationalistic racism of the late nineteenth century which grew out of it. Both forms were replaced in the late nineteenth and early twentieth centuries by the doctrine of "scientific racism" which placed the literary view of racial differences on a supposedly biological foundation, arguing the fixity, definitiveness, and immutability of racial characteristics. Today in America the word "racism" is no longer used popularly to denote theories of racial superiority, but to indicate discrimination against blacks. In this book the term "racist" denotes a proponent of the doctrine of "scientific racism." Such individuals believed in the existence of racial stereotypes, accepted the myth that certain races possess a monopoly of desirable characteristics, and thought that racial differences are caused invariably by heredity, thereby being resistant to any modification or change. Here "racist" refers only to those individuals who had a strong emotional stake in the outcome of studies of racial differences—persons whose acceptance of "Aryan" or "Nordic" superiority was determined mainly by prejudice against non-"Nordics" rather than by an objective analysis of the existing scientific evidence.[4]

Though many eugenicists were "racist," they must be evaluated in relation to the scientific, social, and ethical standards of their own period rather than to those of the present. Living in an age which has followed the Depression and World War II, people today have been influenced by

3. For one of the classic analyses of race from a genetic standpoint, see Boyd, *Genetics*. A historical discussion of the impact of genetics on anthropology is found in T. K. Penniman, *A Hundred Years of Anthropology*, 3rd ed. (London: Gerald Duckworth & Co., 1965), chapter 6.

4. An emotional investment in one's work can be found in thinkers of the political left as well as right. In *The Open and Closed Mind* (New York: Basic Books, 1960), Milton Rokeach points out that the closed mind may be a property of individuals of both political extremes. Nicholas Pastore in *The Nature–Nurture Controversy* (New York: King's Crown Press, 1949) shows social and political conservatism to be correlated with an acceptance of hereditary determinism, liberalism with a belief in the predominance of environment. While the extreme hereditarian interpretation was never without critics, not until the 1930's did it become widely discredited.

environmental explanations of man's social behavior as well as by a popular revulsion against prejudice and theories of racial superiority. However, during the time in which the eugenics movement enjoyed peak influence, in the years between 1905 and 1930, an inflexibly deterministic hereditarian interpretation of human nature was still the dominant view, particularly among the educated. The era was in some ways quite innocent; it did not know the Depression, the second World War, or the atomic bomb. The term "prejudice" lacked the emotional impact which it now possesses. World War II was followed by a widespread abhorrence of prejudice, whereas World War I had been followed by a violent wave of hostility toward minority groups. How greatly the climate of that day differed from that of the present! Though from the standpoint of today the eugenicists appear naive and occasionally sinister, they were the products of their time. In the following pages it is my intention to study the framework in which they made their judgments—often false—in order to understand better the present and prepare for the future.

2

The American Eugenics Movement: 1905–1930

1. Values and Commitments

In 1900, with the rediscovery of Mendel's classic paper of 1866, the science of genetics entered its modern era and began a remarkable development which soon brought it to an eminent position among the sciences. As soon as the science of genetics began, many individuals started speaking of its social import and potential applicability to social problems. Across the world arose organizations devoted to eugenic purposes: in England, the United States, Germany, Scandinavia, Italy, Austria, France, Japan, and in South America. There were national differences among the eugenic societies from the various countries, but all these societies were devoted to the popularization of genetic science, urging that social legislation be guided by what they considered biological wisdom. The epitome of this trend was the American eugenics movement, whose national headquarters was at the Eugenics Record Office at Cold Spring Harbor, Long Island.[1]

From around 1905 to the early 1930's, eugenicists in the United States proposed a two-part policy to upgrade the hereditary quality of the American people. One part they termed "negative eugenics," the elimination of undesired traits from the population by discouraging "unworthy" parenthood. Through appropriate measures—including marriage restriction, sterilization, and permanent custody of defectives—eugenicists hoped to prevent the propagation of epileptics, criminals, alcoholics, the feebleminded, the insane, prostitutes, and others whose physical infirmities or behavioral tendencies they considered to be hereditarily determined. Most eugenicists were so alarmed at what they believed to be a rapid rise in the number of

---

1. For an informative history of the American eugenics movement see Mark H. Haller, *Eugenics: Hereditarian Attitudes in American Thought* (New Brunswick, N.J.: Rutgers University Press, 1963).

defectives that they felt negative eugenic measures must be implemented and enforced by legislation. "Society must protect itself," wrote Charles B. Davenport, a well-known geneticist and the leading American eugenicist of the pre-Depression era, "as it claims the right to deprive the murderer of his life so also it may annihilate the hideous serpent of hopelessly vicious protoplasm."[2]

The other important part of eugenic policy was "positive eugenics," the effort to increase desired traits in the population by encouraging "worthy" parenthood. Since the social and technical difficulties facing positive eugenics were so great, most eugenicists felt no more could be done than to educate the public on the "facts" of heredity in the hope that "superior" couples would voluntarily heed the message to have more children. It was with some dismay that Herbert J. Webber, a well-known plant breeder and eugenicist from Cornell University, wrote: "Positive constructive eugenics is mainly limited to the encouragement that can be given to the production of large families among the better classes."[3] Some eugenicists were quite pessimistic and felt that the implementation of "positive" programs was a hopelessly discouraging task to which even "eugenic education" could make little contribution. One well-known eugenicist declared: "The geneticist can only point out the problem and emphasize as much as possible the urgency of its solution. Unless economic and social changes permit and encourage people of superior morality and intelligence to have more children, eugenics can make little progress."[4]

Curiously, this two-part plan of "positive" and "negative" eugenics constituted the eugenics movement's official program for the entire period from the turn of the century until the early years of the Depression. This was true of eugenics not only in America but elsewhere as well. The participants at the Third International Eugenics Congress (New York, 1932) believed in the basic validity of this program as much as the delegates at the First International Eugenics Congress (London, 1912)[5] –

2. Charles B. Davenport, "Report of Committee on Eugenics," *American Breeders' Magazine*, 1(1910):129.
3. Herbert J. Webber, "Eugenics from the Point of View of the Geneticist," in *Eugenics: Twelve University Lectures* (New York: Dodd, Mead, and Co., 1914), p. 143.
4. Paul Popenoe, "Will Morality Disappear?" *Journal of Heredity*, 9(October, 1918):270.
5. The proceedings of these congresses were published as *Problems in Eugenics.* Papers Communicated to the First International Eugenics Congress (London: Eugenics Education Society, 1912); and *A Decade of Progress in Eugenics.* Scientific Papers of the Third International Congress of Eugenics (Baltimore: Williams and Wilkins Co., 1934).

despite the fact that the interim between these two congresses witnessed the development of the theory of the gene, the elucidation of the physical basis of inheritance, the demonstration that mutations of the gene can be artificially produced by irradiation, and the development of population genetics into a sophisticated science, not to mention important advances in psychology and anthropology. Throughout this period, of course, eugenicists debated the particulars of the eugenics program. Some thought that war served as a "eugenic" agent by allowing the strong to kill off the weak;[6] others contended that war was "dysgenic," permitting the weak to destroy the strong. Similarly, eugenicists argued whether birth control was "dysgenic" or "eugenic," that is, whether the measure would be employed more by "superior" or "inferior" persons. But despite their continual examination of the details of the eugenics program, most eugenicists never examined the deeper ethical and scientific assumptions of the movement. Few eugenicists ever bothered to consider such troublesome matters as whether their breeding programs could be justified technologically in the light of recent findings in genetics or whether men really possess the wisdom to decide which traits are desirable.

The American eugenics movement was intellectually static, virtually unchanging in its membership and leadership. The hierarchy of the movement was self-perpetuating and entrenched. In the 1930's most of the movement's leaders—Charles Davenport, Harry H. Laughlin, Henry F. Osborn, David Starr Jordan, Paul Popenoe, Madison Grant, and others— were those who had helped organize the movement twenty-five years earlier. Rosters of officers of various eugenic societies in the late 1920's and 1930's showed few names which had not been involved for the preceding twenty years. Eugenics thus was failing to attract the younger generation. To understand why the American eugenics movement became static, it is necessary to examine its origins.

Though the idea of improving the hereditary quality of the human race dates back as far as Plato's *Republic*, the modern concept of eugenics began to be discussed during the second half of the nineteenth century. Underlying the early modern interest in eugenics was a philosophical belief among many in the notion of human perfectibility. Even in the eighteenth century such thinkers as Voltaire, Rousseau, and Condorcet had advanced this notion, and throughout the nineteenth century Western Man continued to pay homage to that ideal. The Industrial Revolution, in emanci-

6. Most American eugenicists who believed war to be "eugenic" were not sympathetic to totalitarianism; nevertheless, some Nazis used that same argument to justify Germany's bombing of Spain during the Spanish Civil War.

pating humanity from an agricultural existence, undoubtedly helped foster an early attitude of optimism, of hope for a golden future, of human perfectibility in the consumption of material goods.[7]

In 1848 John Humphrey Noyes, a Perfectionist preacher, was the first in modern times to suggest the possibility of improving the human race specifically by judicious breeding. After the theory of evolution had been promulgated, Francis Galton, an English gentleman of wide scientific interests and a cousin of Charles Darwin, became the leading advocate of eugenic programs in the English-speaking world. As early as 1865 it was his view that "if a twentieth part of the cost and pains were spent in measures for the improvement of the human race that is spent on the improvement of the breed of horses and cattle, what a galaxy of genius might we not create."[8] By the mid-1880's the term "eugenics," which Galton had coined, had become commonplace.

Galton's ideas were a logical outgrowth of the theory of evolution and enjoyed a degree of currency at a time when it became increasingly popular to apply the doctrine of evolution to non-biological situations. Darwin himself was reluctant to discuss publicly the non-scientific implications of evolution, but others were not.[9] One result of this trend, representing the

7. Such was the concern with well-being in the nineteenth century that even so unlikely a figure as Marx in his doctoral thesis investigated the matter!

8. Francis Galton, "Hereditary Talent and Character," *MacMillan's Magazine*, 12(1865):165.

Galton's life and work are the subject of Karl Pearson, *The Life and Labours of Francis Galton*, 3 vols. in 4 (Cambridge: Cambridge University Press, 1914–30). Ruth Schwartz Cowan examines the relation between Galton's scientific work and his social philosophy in "Sir Francis Galton and the Study of Heredity in the Nineteenth Century" (Johns Hopkins University, unpublished Doctoral Dissertation, 1969). How ironic that Galton, the founder of eugenics, was himself childless!

9. Darwin himself was aware of many of the broader implications of his theory. A pious and devout youth who had intended to enter the ministry, his study of evolution drove him away from religion until he finally rejected Christianity and belief in a Creator. What evidently shattered Darwin's faith was the chance and evil he observed in the biological world. "I cannot persuade myself," he wrote, "that a beneficient and omnipotent God would have designedly created the Ichneumonidae with the express intention of their feeding within the living bodies of caterpillars, or that cats should play with mice." (Charles Darwin to Asa Gray, 22 May 1860, in Francis Darwin, ed., *The Autobiography of Charles Darwin and Selected Letters* [New York: Dover Publications, 1958], p. 249.) Professor Donald Fleming has suggested, however, that while Darwin was aware of such implications of evolution, he was chary to discuss them in detail publicly; in a tactical maneuver designed to win adherents to his theory, he tended to play down its unorthodox implications. While his private correspondence, especially after 1861, suggests that Darwin dropped the idea of a Creator, in his published writings he continued to make gestures of appeasement to the religious, insisting that evolution was compatible with theism and that evolution meant God was not less wonderful but more so. Darwin continually emphasized that the theory was not concerned with accounting for the ultimate origins

major impact of evolution upon intellectual thought, was the development of "naturalism." Naturalism included a number of ideas, the most important of which were a veneration of scientific fact at the most dependable form of knowledge, confidence in the analogy between human society and biological organisms, the belief that societies progress in distinct epochs or cultural stages, and the notion that the rate at which a society or part of a society changes depends on its proximity to technological advances. By the 1870's naturalism had developed a strong grip on the American mind, an effect felt especially by the intelligentsia.[10]

No part of the naturalistic world-view enjoyed greater influence in America during the late nineteenth and early twentieth centuries than the analogy between society and biological organisms, an idea which was advanced by Herbert Spencer and which sometimes went by the name "Social Darwinism." So strong was Spencer's hold on the American mind that in 1905 Associate Justice Oliver Wendell Holmes, Jr., felt constrained to remind his colleagues on the United States Supreme Court that Spencer was *not* part of the United States Constitution.[11] Between the 1860's and 1903, the sale of Spencer's works in America came close to 400,000 volumes, an extraordinary total for books on such technical subjects as philosophy and sociology; and during these years scholars in all fields had to come to terms with Spencer's views.[12]

Social Darwinism was based upon the principle of evolution as universal law. According to this doctrine, evolution applies not only to life but to the physical cosmos and human societies as well. Spencer felt that evolution involves the development of the homogeneous to the heterogeneous, the undifferentiated to the differentiated, the unintegrated to the integrated. He imagined the origin and development of society in the following way: at first, isolated individuals performing simple tasks without specialization; ultimately, an order more diverse, specialized, and interdependent. In this system, the principle of individualism was powerful. While society

---

of species, only for changes which had occurred among organisms once life had been created. He also tended to shy away from the issue of the evolution of man, making his first complete statement on the matter only in 1871 in *Descent of Man*. To win the scientific acceptance of his theory, Darwin fastidiously seemed to avoid non-scientific controversy. (Professor Donald Fleming, lectures in "The History of Science in America," Harvard University.)

10. For a discussion of naturalism the reader is referred to the unit on "The Naturalistic Mind, 1865–1929" in Stow Persons, *American Minds. A History of Ideas* (New York: Henry Holt and Co., 1958).

11. See Holmes's dissenting opinion in Lochner v. New York, 198 U.S. 45 (1905).

12. Richard Hofstadter, *Social Darwinism in American Thought*, rev. ed. (Boston: Beacon Press, 1955), p. 34. This book remains the outstanding interpretation of the impact of Social Darwinism on American life.

grew more complex with progress, it also became freer and more diverse, and hence the evolution of the individual was toward greater freedom and less constraint. Competition was regarded as the key to progress. Social Darwinists were against any attempt on the part of government to legislate social reform; they felt government welfare programs represented an infraction of individual liberty and, by favoring the "unfit," interfered with the process of human evolution. Spencer facilely identified the "unfit" with the poor, whom he felt may safely be left to die out. Social Darwinism thus represented a major attempt to apply the methods and discoveries of biology to the analysis of non-scientific issues, an ideal which profoundly influenced the intellectuals of that generation. Spencer himself remarked, "My ultimate purpose, lying behind all proximate purposes, has been that of finding for the principles of right and wrong in conduct at large, a scientific basis."[13]

In the 1870's and 1880's, despite its great popularity in the United States, Social Darwinism was not without its critics, and at no time did it enjoy an uncontested hold over the American mind. Certain intellectuals maintained, contrary to the views of Social Darwinists, that there exists a qualitative difference between man's social and physical evolution, a position which justified their faith in education and charity as devices to help uplift the unfortunate. The leading advocate of this position in the United States was Lester F. Ward, the earliest American sociologist of importance. Even Darwin and Wallace, the co-architects of the theory of evolution, rejected Spencer's social interpretations! A Fabian Socialist, Wallace believed that land should be nationalized and opportunity equalized in order that selection could operate most efficiently. Darwin, a humane man, voiced disgust with slavery and would have been shocked to hear evolutionary theory used to justify the subjugation and "inferiority" of the Negro.[14]

Nevertheless, throughout the 1870's and 1880's Social Darwinism exerted enormous influence in America. In the rugged, individualistic Spencerian interpretation of evolution, many Americans saw the image of their own society. America was growing rapidly, both geographically and technologically, and its exploitive methods, fierce competition, and disdain for failure seemed to resemble closely the popular picture of Darwinian exist-

13. Herbert Spencer, *The Data of Ethics* (New York: D. Appleton and Co., 1879), p. v.
14. See Wilma George, *Biologist Philosopher: A Study of the Life and Writings of Alfred Russel Wallace* (London: Abelard-Schuman, 1964), *passim*; and Francis Darwin, ed., *The Life and Letters of Charles Darwin*, vol. 2 (London: John Murray, 1887), pp. 246, 248, and 341.

ence. Business entrepreneurs and unprincipled politicians seemed instinctively to be attracted by the "survival philosophy." So did a middle class inspired by the dream of personal conquest and individual assertion. In addition, Social Darwinism could be used to buttress the prevailing political mood of the era, which, because of rapid economic change and weariness with the antebellum political agitation, was generally conservative. Its catchwords of "survival of the fittest" and "struggle for existence" gave biological force to the notions that nature allows only its "fittest" members to survive and that such competition results in social progress. Moreover, the concept of geologic time intrinsic to evolutionary theory supported the conservative notion that change must be unhurried. Viewing society as an organism, one could envision constructive change occurring only at the same slow pace at which organisms evolve. The Spencerian interpretation of evolution was thus not a necessary one, only a possible one, a fact which suggests that social and intellectual commitments might sometimes be more important than truth and logic in determining which social ideas were accepted.

Before 1900, despite the popularity of the naturalistic viewpoint and the urgings of Francis Galton, an organized eugenics crusade did not develop in the United States. A number of eugenic societies were established in the late nineteenth century, most notably Loring Moody's Institute of Heredity in Boston (1880), but none of these survived for long or engendered much popular enthusiasm. At this time the lack of knowledge about the process of inheritance impeded the growth of a eugenics movement in America. Nothing was known of the physical basis of heredity; chromosomes were discovered in the nucleus only in the 1880's, and it was not until the turn of the century that their function as the carriers of the genes was detected. In addition, biologists had no rule governing the transmission of traits from one generation to the next; the only guidelines they had were the vague notion employed by breeders that "like produces like" and the principle that all traits represent a "blend" of parental characteristics. Finally, popular belief in the inheritance of acquired characteristics made eugenic proposals seem unnecessary to many, since this theory belied the notion that improvements in the hereditary endowment of man could result only from breeding programs.

With the birth of modern genetics, these undercurrents of interest in eugenics were transformed into a stable, institutionalized movement. In providing a long-sought explanation for the transmission and distribution of traits from one generation to the next, Mendel's laws enabled eugenic proposals to be appreciated on a heretofore impossible scale. Eugenic breeding programs now became widely appealing because at last they could be based upon biological theory rather than upon the imprecise rules used by breeders. "Mendel gave it [the eugenics program] its biological mechanisms and experimental method,"[15] one eugenicist remarked. The popularization after 1900 of the work of August Weismann, who disproved the theory that acquired characteristics can be inherited, helped intensify interest in a eugenics movement. The sentiment for a eugenics movement had already been present before 1900; the rise of genetics allowed this sentiment to be mobilized.

Thus, at the turn of the century both the general social and intellectual atmosphere of the day and those scientific developments which resulted in the birth of genetics as a discipline helped create interest for a eugenics movement. Because eugenicists comprised a diverse group of individuals from a wide range of professional activities, however, some responded more to one than to the other influence. Many geneticists, for example, were prompted to join the movement early in the century by the biological developments, though the social-intellectual milieu also contributed to their interest. Nevertheless, at a time when many Americans were preoccupied with what they considered to be a sharply rising increase in physical and mental degeneracy in the country, when many feared that civilization was interfering with the working of natural selection, most were interested in eugenics primarily because it offered a "scientific" solution compatible with the world view of the naturalistic mind. In what was only an exaggeration of a very common tendency of the day, eugenicists regarded the scientific method with reverence, trusting completely its ability to analyze social problems and to prescribe behavior. One not untypical eugenicist regarded "the laboratory" as "the new Mount Sinai" and spoke of "the Ten Commandments of Science."[16] They found the idea of a eugenics movement attractive because it provided pressing social "problems" with a biological solution.

Ironically, though eugenicists revered the scientific method, few ever bothered to master the methods and knowledge of the science upon which their social programs were allegedly based. Of the more than one hundred individuals who served on the Advisory Council of the American Eugenics Society in the 1920's, about ten per cent were trained geneticists. A small circular, *What I Think About Eugenics*, contained statements by 143 leading American eugenicists, of whom only eight were trained in genetics or biology. Popular works on eugenics usually began with expositions of "genetic science," but these discussions of heredity usually showed little

15. Albert E. Wiggam, *The New Decalogue of Science* (Indianapolis: Bobbs-Merrill Co., 1923), p. 99.
16. *Ibid.*, pp. 79, 99.

understanding of the subject. One author was honest enough to preface his book by boasting to the reader that he had "avoided even reading books on heredity."[17] In general these men were sincere and well-intentioned, but their claim that the eugenic program rested firmly upon a valid genetic foundation was based more on faith than on first-hand assurance. To most of them, eugenics assumed the proportions not of a science but of a social crusade. One eugenicist spoke of "the nobility of the ideal which it involves";[18] another claimed that "Eugenics is the reform that underlies, creates and preserves all other reforms."[19] For three decades the social climate in America permitted that crusade to flourish. It mattered little that genetic science progressed rapidly during those thirty years, for eugenicists tended to understand the later developments no better than they did the initial discoveries in genetics that for a short time made eugenic schemes seem feasible. Even though some geneticists in the 1920's were grumbling about eugenicists' use of "genetics" to justify their programs, American society at large was still receptive to a discussion of eugenic ideas. In light of these facts, one can begin to understand eugenicists' long, rigid adherence to one theme.

The inflexible and static qualities of American eugenics are only partially explained by the commitment of most eugenicists to the movement as a social crusade. For a fuller explanation, the eugenicists must be compared with another group of early twentieth-century American reformers, the progressives. The "progressive movement" was that upsurge of reform sentiment and activity in which respectable middle-class citizens turned their attention and energies toward correcting the social, political, and economic ills they saw in society. The progressives fought corruption and inefficiency in all levels of government, expressed indignation over the power of the political machines and of big business, and attended to the problems of the poor, the slums, and social injustice. A strong sense of moral purpose pervaded the movement, and many contemporary writers interpret it as an effort to recapture the morality and civic purity which were commonly believed to have been lost during the processes of industrialization and urbanization.[20]

17. W. E. D. Stokes, *The Right to be Well-Born* (New York: C. J. O'Brien, 1917), p. 141.

18. Albert G. Keller, "Eugenics and its Social Limitations," in *Eugenics: Twelve University Lectures*, p. 240.

19. Statement by Daniel W. LaRue in *What I Think About Eugenics*, bound between pp. 8 and 9, in Eugenics Society of the United States of America, *A Brief Bibliography of Eugenics* (n.p., 192–), p. [8].

20. The outstanding interpretation not only of the progressives but of the entire reform impulse in America is Richard Hofstadter's *The Age of Reform* (New York: Alfred Knopf, 1955).

In a recent book Donald Pickens pointed out that both the eugenicists and the progressives were strongly influenced by the naturalistic tradition of the late nineteenth century and that many progressives endorsed eugenic proposals for uplifting the race.[21] It may be added to Pickens' observations that sociologically the eugenicists and progressives represented similar groups and that a large number of eugenicists also supported many progressive reforms. Eugenicists, like the progressives, came in largest numbers from the native-born, Anglo-Saxon, Protestant, upper middle class and formed part of that generation's educators, scientists, scholars, journalists, physicians, lawyers, and clergy. All parts of the country were represented in the eugenics movement, though the East and Northeast were by far the largest contributors.[22] Eugenicists came from both the city and the countryside, even though the great majority, including most of the city dwellers among them, shared the progressive's fear of the "corrupting" influence of urban life. "Cities are consumers of men and the country side producers of them," one New York City eugenicist wrote. "So we still have a chance for the future if we are able to keep the blood of the countrymen pure."[23]

Most eugenicists sympathized with progressive goals, many even regarding themselves as progressive reformers. Some eugenicists employed progressive jargon in their writings. In one widely read popular treatise on eugenics, for instance, the author argued for the "use of trained analytical intelligence"[24] in government and complained that "government and social control are in the hands of expert politicians who have power,

21. Donald K. Pickens, *Eugenics and the Progressives* (Nashville: Vanderbilt University Press, 1968).
22. An analysis of the backgrounds of the 144 leading eugenicists who contributed to the pamphlet *What I Think About Eugenics* provides the following statistics:

Occupation		Geographical Area Represented	
Educator	47	West	24
Scientist	22	Midwest	24
Clergy	19	South	20
Professor (lib. art)	16	East-Northeast	68
Physician	10	Undetermined	8
Author-Journalist	8		
Politician	5		
Lawyer	4		
Philanthropist	2		
Banker-Businessman	2		
Other	9		

23. Madison Grant to Rupert F. Hall, March 3, 1913, *IRL*.
24. Wiggam, *New Decalogue*, p. 276.

instead of expert technologists who have wisdom. There should be technologists in control of every field of human need and desire."[25] Prominent
eugenicists often participated in such typically progressive endeavors as the
conservation movement, the Boy Scouts, and the efforts to improve city
and local government.[26] Madison Grant, John C. Merriam, and Henry F.
Osborn, all well-known eugenicists, were leading conservationists and
friends of Theodore Roosevelt; David Starr Jordan, chairman of the
Eugenics Committee of the American Breeders' Association, served as
national vice president of the Boy Scouts. The University of Wisconsin's
popular and controversial sociologist, Edward A. Ross, best exemplified
this pattern. As a member of the Advisory Council of the American
Eugenics Society, a staunch supporter of compulsory sterilization
measures and of birth control, and the author of a widely read plea for
immigration restriction, *The Old World in the New* (1914), Ross's position
of leadership within the eugenics movement was unquestioned. His muck-
raking, his involvement with Robert La Follette's University of Wisconsin
braintrust (how "wonderfully pleasant" was "the political atmosphere of
Wisconsin," he remarked, "after the great clean-up led by the virile La
Follette"[27]), his vigorous defenses of academic freedom, and his leadership
in the American Association of University Professors had also made him an
eminent progressive. Like some progressives from rural areas, he also possessed a deeply ingrained abhorrence of alcohol. His feelings on the matter
were so great that he once found geneticist Raymond Pearl's "frivolous
attitude toward the drink habit" a sufficient reason to distrust some of
Pearl's scientific work.[28]

Eugenicists shared the progressives' concern with moral intangibles. To
most eugenicists, the movement was not just a social crusade but a moral
crusade as well. They so venerated science and the scientific method that
they came to regard the acceptance of eugenic programs as a religious duty
imposed by the theory of evolution, many of them even calling the movement a secular religion. In this outlook they were greatly influenced by
Galton, who was the first to speak of eugenics in this way. In 1883 he had
written:

> The chief result of these Inquiries has been to elicit the religious signif-
> icance of the doctrine of evolution. It suggests an alteration in our mental
> attitude, and imposes a new moral duty. The new mental attitude is one of

25. *Ibid.*, p. 277.
26. Note that the movements of eugenics, conservation, and child welfare shared
the common theme of "preserving natural resources."
27. Edward A. Ross, *Seventy Years of It* (New York: D. Appleton-Century Co.,
1936), p. 293.
28. Edward A. Ross to Mrs. Anita Newcomb McGee, May 15, 1928, *EAR*.

a greater sense of moral freedom, responsibility, and opportunity; the new duty which is supposed to be exercised concurrently with, and not in opposition to the old ones upon which the social fabric depends, is an endeavour to further evolution, especially that of the human race.[29]

In this tradition, American eugenicists spoke of "the religion of evolution,"[30] "the duty of upbuilding the human race,"[31] and "the moral implication in the doctrine of evolution."[32] They let science act as a constraint upon their actions; they allowed science to tell them that individual desires are less important than the biological and moral imperative of improving the human race; they permitted biology to assume religion's traditional function of defining permissible conduct. It was their view that "in no other line can science and religion so closely cooperate as in the production of races of strong people."[33]

Eugenicists evinced their concern for moral intangibles in their consideration of eugenics as the key not only to the physical betterment of mankind but also to the *intellectual* and *moral* advancement of the race. As one eugenicist put it, "Biological facts clearly indicate that only through the application of eugenic measures can man reach a permanently higher plane of intellect and morals."[34] Resident Bishop F. D. Leete of the Methodist Church in Indianapolis believed that "unless eugenical principles are put into effect" it will be "impossible for good government, civilization and Christianity to achieve their ideals."[35] Another eugenicist declared, "*Moral Education* is the procedure by which the achievement of personality and institutional progress are promoted. Race Betterment means just that."[36] Eugenicists' strong feeling of moral purpose understandably contributed to their marked self-assuredness and sense of self-righteousness in discussing the eugenic program.

The devotion of most eugenicists to the moral crusade of eugenics was limitless. Ross felt that "interest in eugenics is almost a perfect index of one's breadth of outlook and unselfish concern for the future of our

29. Francis Galton, *Inquiries into Human Faculty and its Development* (New York: Macmillan and Co., 1883), p. 337.

30. E. G. Conklin, *The Direction of Human Evolution* (New York: Charles Scribner's Sons, 1921), p. 237.

31. Statement by Sidney Cazort in *What I Think About Eugenics*, p. [6].

32. C. E. Rugh, "Moral Education," in *Proceedings of the Third Race Betterment Conference* (Battle Creek, Michigan: The Race Betterment Foundation, 1928), p. 672.

33. "Narrow Limits for Breeding Men," *American Breeders' Magazine*, 1(April-June, 1910):144.

34. Statement by Charles F. Dight in *What I Think About Eugenics*, p. [8].

35. Statement by F. D. Leete, *ibid.*, p. [3].

36. Rugh, "Moral Education," p. 681.

race."[37] Irving Fisher, a Yale University economist, wrote: "I believe that eugenics is incomparably the greatest concern of the human race."[38] The dedication of the eugenicists was in one sense the strength of the movement. When they campaigned for legislation, officials and other citizens could not help but heed the fervent, impassioned pleas of so many eminent persons. Eugenicists' conviction, on the other hand, was also the fatal weakness of the movement, for many eugenicists possessed a moral absolutism so strong that they lost the ability to distinguish reality from fantasy. Though the United States census of 1920 for the first time showed the city population to exceed the rural population, one eugenicist at a conference in *1928* made the astounding claim that "rural districts supply a disproportionately large part of the future population," predicting further that in four generations the rural stock would constitute eighty-eight per cent of the total population![39] Entertaining few doubts about the efficacy of their programs, eugenicists tended to assume that eugenic measures would be employed universally once the public was informed of the "facts" of heredity. Even so rational and moderate a eugenicist as Lewellys F. Barker, Professor of Medicine at Johns Hopkins, believed that "when people are made familiar with the facts [of heredity], they will, themselves, find the way practically to apply them."[40] Many eugenicists, in short, were so imbued with moral righteousness that they often seemed blind to some of the insuperable difficulties they faced. It was as if they felt they already possessed the "Truth" and saw little need to re-examine their assumptions.

Thus, the eugenics movement throughout its entire existence did not modify its basic goals or program. This situation resulted from the tendency of eugenicists to regard the movement as a social and moral crusade and from the strength of their commitment to naturalistic assumptions about man and society. In reviewing the movement one is left with a realization of the fundamental paradoxes in eugenicists' world view: their worship of science and their sophomoric understanding of the genetic framework upon which they based their programs; their appeal to reason and education in trying to promote the popular acceptance of eugenic ideology and their own passionate, irrational commitment to the eugenic program; their conviction of the soundness of the Social Darwinistic principles of laissez faire and individualism and their advocacy of state control

37. Statement by Edward A. Ross in *What I Think About Eugenics*, p. [3].
38. Statement by Irving Fisher, *ibid.*, p. [5].
39. Luther S. West, "The Practical Application of Eugenic Principles," in *Proceedings of the Third Race Betterment Conference*, p. 92.
40. Lewellys F. Barker, "Foreword," in *Eugenics: Twelve University Lectures*, p. xiii.

as a means by which to achieve eugenic goals. The majority of eugenicists did not change their views with the times, nor did they realize the inconsistencies of their position, and in the end they committed acts which to the present-day historian seem foolish; but it is important to understand the spirit in which those things were done.

2. The Restrictionists

Though most eugenicists were sincere and well-intentioned, they were also biased since they tended to approach the eugenics crusade with the presuppositions of the conservative upper and upper middle classes. It was not uncommon to find eugenicists scorning the masses ("our idiotic public,"[41] as eugenicist Prescott F. Hall described them), and they commonly felt, as another put it, that the upper classes "contain much of the best [hereditary] ability in our population."[42] Even Davenport, Director of the Eugenics Record Office and the acknowledged leader of American eugenicists, equated the lower class with inferior genes;[43] and others went so far as to eulogize the upper classes, claiming that these groups were responsible for virtually all of human progress.[44] Some eugenicists, not surprisingly, showed a fascination and admiration for what they considered to be the notability of their own ancestry. Jordan wrote, "The assumption, well justified by facts, is that revolutionary fathers were a superior type of men, and that to have had such names in our personal ancestry [as Jordan had in his] is of itself a cause for thinking more highly of ourselves."[45] "Any healthy New England family," he said also, "which can show its connection with England can also show its connection with most of the nobility of England, and with royal families of all the world except China and Patagonia."[46]

In entertaining these presuppositions, eugenicists were reflecting the cultural consciousness of the period, not of themselves alone. As well-to-do members of society, they had vested interests in propound-

41. Prescott F. Hall to E. A. Ross, October 18, 1914, *EAR.*
42. Warren S. Thompson, "Race Suicide in the United States," *American Journal of Physical Anthropology*, 3(1920):146.
43. See Charles B. Davenport, *Heredity in Relation to Eugenics* (New York: Henry Holt and Co., 1911), pp. 8, 80.
44. See, for example, Frederick Adams Woods, *The Influence of Monarchs* (New York: Macmillan, 1913), p. 422.
45. David Starr Jordan, *The Human Harvest: A Study of the Decay of Races Through the Survival of the Unfit* (Boston: American Unitarian Association, 1907), p. 104.
46. David Starr Jordan to Charles B. Davenport, March 20, 1911, *CBD.*

ing the genetic superiority of these groups, but large numbers of non-eugenicists also felt the same way. Such views could readily be justified at a time in American history when the business, intellectual, and cultural leaders still arose almost exclusively from an old-stock upper class which was white, Anglo-Saxon, and Protestant.[47] In the late nineteenth and early twentieth centuries, even those most vigorous defenders of equal opportunity for immigrants—the social workers—tended to be haughty, self-righteous, and conscious of their own "superiority." They usually entered the slums with honorable intentions and lofty ideals, but very often their effectiveness was diminished by their Anglo-Saxon values, inability to understand the problems of the poor, and condescension quite noticeable to their clients.[48]

Eugenicists possessed a racial as well as a class bias: they were evolutionists who regarded the Anglo-Saxon or "Nordic" type they saw dominating world affairs as nature's "fittest race." Of course, race and caste prejudice did not begin with the eugenicists but has been known throughout history in virtually all societies. Indeed, there is evidence that race prejudice existed in India as long as five thousand years ago.[49] In the nineteenth century, nevertheless, racial prejudice began to inspire sophisticated theories of racial superiority. Several writers of that period, most notably Count Arthur de Gobineau of France, Houston Stewart Chamberlain of England, and William Z. Ripley of the United States, articulated theories which gained especially wide currency in the Western world and which later provided eugenicists the foundations of their racial views. Gobineau authored a four-volume *Essay on the Inequality of Races* (1853-55) in which he attempted to prove that the ills which had befallen France since the Revolution stemmed from the racial mongrelization of the previously pure Teutonic nobility. In *Foundations of the Nineteenth Century* (1899), Chamberlain, son-in-law of the chauvinistic German composer Richard Wagner, attributed Germany's greatness to the fact that only Teutons possess the capability for military, political, cultural, and scientific distinction. Ripley was not a racist (he attributed racial differences to social conditions and geography as well as to heredity), but his *The Races of Europe* (1899) provided the anthropological division of

47. For an analysis of the role of caste in American history see E. Digby Baltzell, *The Protestant Establishment; Aristocracy and Caste in America* (New York: Random House, 1964).
48. See Oscar Handlin's remarks on the first generation social worker in *The Uprooted* (New York: Grosset and Dunlap, 1951), pp. 280–82.
49. See the chapter on "Early Race Theories" in Thomas F. Gossett, *Race: The History of an Idea in America* (Dallas: Southern Methodist University Press, 1963).

Europeans into three races which most anthropologists and eugenicists quickly adopted.[50]

Though such theories existed long before the eugenics movement, eugenicists expanded these early ideas and cast them into an evolutionary framework. Following a common misinterpretation of Darwinism, they postulated a unilinear vertical progression from the lowest to the highest.[51] They considered the Negro race biologically inferior to the Mongoloid race, which they in turn deemed inferior to the exalted Caucasian race. Within the white race they felt there existed a three-fold classification consisting of the "Mediterraneans," the "Alpines," and the "Nordics." According to this scheme, the Mediterraneans, who populated southern Europe, were a dolichocephalic (long-skulled) race of dark complexion and short, slight stature. The Alpines, a brachycephalic (round-skulled) people of medium height, sturdy build, and intermediate complexion, inhabited the central and eastern regions of Europe. In the northern parts of Europe lived the long-skulled Nordics, a very tall race of blue-eyed blondes. Nordics were Protestant; Alpines and Mediterraneans were Catholic. In general, eugenicists believed that the "Nordic" race possessed a monopoly of desirable characteristics, physical and mental, thereby standing as the superior race. They regarded these racial traits to be firmly and immutably established by heredity, insensitive to change or modification through environmental influences. The leading expositor of this position among eugenicists, Madison Grant, thus compared such typical Nordic *racial* characteristics as "love of organization, of law and military efficiency, as well as the ideals of family life, loyalty, and

50. These men are discussed by Gossett, *ibid.* European race theories are also examined in Jacques Barzun, *Race: A Study in Modern Superstition* (New York: Harcourt, Brace and Co., 1937); and T. K. Penniman, *A Hundred Years of Anthropology*, 3rd ed. (London: Gerald Duckworth & Co., 1965).

51. Many interpreters of Darwin correctly accepted the idea of *change* implicit to evolution but mistook all change to be *linear*. Such persons failed to realize that the terminal twigs of a taxonomic system cannot readily be classified into a linear, historical sequence. During Darwin's generation and for a time afterwards, these erroneous applications of evolutionary thought to a broad range of situations were well-known and widely accepted. In addition to the view of race described here, there were two other especially popular interpretations of evolution. One was the theory, proclaimed by Lewis Henry Morgan in 1877, that there exists a universally valid sequence of seven stages in the development of all human societies. According to this view, no society can pass through a unique cultural stage. The second was the doctrine of recapitulation, which maintained that during fetal development the embryo successively passes through the adult stages of the organisms which preceded it in evolution (or, as Ernst Haeckel aphorized, "ontology recapitulates phylogeny"). This theory once reached the status of a fundamental biogenetic law. Darwin himself accepted the doctrine of embryological recapitulation, though not that of races or of cultures.

truth"[52] with what he considered such representative Mediterranean racial traits as a "volatile and analytical spirit, lack of cohesion, political incapacity, and ready resort to treason."[53] It was his belief that "the amount of Nordic blood in each nation is a very fair measure of its strength in war and standing in civilization."[54]

To eugenicists this view sufficiently explained the achievements of American civilization. They considered the United States fundamentally Nordic in its origin and evolution, and they attributed the country's rapid development to its superior racial components. Believing that the more desirable qualities of Nordics "have little part in the resultant mixture"[55] of Nordics and non-Nordics, eugenicists regarded the greatest danger to the Nordic race to be interbreeding. In order to preserve the superior racial quality of the American people, it became an important feature of "negative eugenics" to urge that immigration to the country be limited to those of Nordic stock. Grant predicted that if the United States did not establish immigration quotas favoring Nordics, the result would be "many amazing racial hybrids and some ethnic horrors that will be beyond the powers of future anthropologists to unravel."[56]

For a time, particularly between 1919 and 1929, this view of race had a strong emotional appeal to many Americans. Despite their confident assertions of the "superiority" of the social elite, many of the old-stock upper class had come to feel increasingly threatened by the masses of immigrants which had poured into the country since the Civil War. In the face of this rising tide of immigrant power, more and more native Americans began to fear that their traditional leadership, prestige, and position were in jeopardy. At the turn of the century the conservative and propertied classes still enjoyed great position and influence. Nevertheless, having just witnessed such displays of social unrest as the Haymarket Riot, the writings of Edward Bellamy, the campaigns of Henry George, the Homestead Strike, the Pullman Strike, Coxey's Army, the Panic of 1893, the Populist Revolt, and the Bryan campaign of 1896, they were engulfed by an attitude of alarm and apprehension. As the challenge of the newcomer increased, the response of many native Americans was that of withdrawal. The late nineteenth century witnessed the beginning of social discrimination in America and the rise of "society" to exclude the new. At that

52. Madison Grant, *The Passing of the Great Race* (New York: Charles Scribner's Sons, 1916), p. 139.
53. *Ibid.*, p. 140.
54. *Ibid.*, p. 175.
55. *Ibid.*, p. 82.
56. *Ibid.*, p. 81.

time arose private boarding schools to rear children "properly" (and to spare them contact with the unseemly newcomers in the heterogeneous public schools), as well as exclusive neighborhoods, country clubs, metropolitan men's clubs, summer resorts, and the definition of aristocracy by ancestry and association rather than by wealth.[57] In 1887 the first Social Register was published, and the 1890's saw a flowering of hereditary and patriotic societies. By 1900 there were seventy such societies in the United States, thirty-five of which had been organized during the preceding decade. These organizations served a useful psychological function for the patrician, since they provided "Americans" a sense of special belonging by virtue of hereditary associations, a certain security from the onslaught and challenge of the new arrivals.[58] Social discrimination became intimately linked with nativism, for this was a period when "respectable" citizens showed a concern with caste, race, and ancestry to an extent which has not been seen in America before or since. Edward A. Ross believed that respect for race and ancestry was requisite for survival in a people.[59] The socially prominent Grant argued that "race feeling might seem like prejudice to those cramped by it, but it is really a natural antipathy which functions to maintain purity of type in a people."[60] The publisher of the Social Register also handled much of the literature of the American Pro-

57. Metropolitan men's clubs had been in existence since the 1830's (the Philadelphia Club, the oldest in America, was established in 1834), but only in the 1880's did they begin excluding prospective members on ethnic grounds. Jess Seligman, for example, who had helped organize New York's Union League during the Civil War, resigned from the club in 1893 after his son had been blackballed for being a Jew. Although a few boarding schools, such as Andover and Exeter, date far back in American history, the boarding school movement also underwent its most rapid growth in the half century after 1880. The remaining social institutions of the aristocracy were created after 1880. See Baltzell, *Protestant Establishment*, chapter 5.

58. These organizations are discussed in Wallace E. Davies, *Patriotism on Parade; The Story of Veterans' and Hereditary Organizations in America 1783-1900* (Cambridge: Harvard University Press, 1955). Hysteria against immigrants, Catholics, and Jews—but not Negroes—prompted the creation of these societies. It seems to me that the reason for this is that Negroes at that time did not constitute a major economic or social threat. Perhaps it is reasonable to suggest that prejudice against non-black minorities at the turn of the century was something like anti-Negro hostility today, now that the black man has become a far stronger economic force. In this regard, Baltzell (*Protestant Establishment*, p. 121) points out what strikes me as an interesting historical parallel. Just as today, when middle class white families of diverse ethnic backgrounds are rapidly escaping from the increasingly Negro composition of the cities, so did the Protestant upper class at the turn of the century begin fleeing from the urban melting pot comprised of immigrants, Catholics, and Jews.

59. Edward A. Ross, *The Old World in the New* (New York: Century Co., 1914), p. 304.

60. Grant, *Passing of the Great Race*, p. 193.

tective Association, which in the 1890's participated heavily in the nativist movement, standing as an early advocate of immigration restriction.[61] After World War I, hereditary and patriotic societies were to be among the most vocal advocates of halting immigration. Eugenicists thus belonged to a generation of Americans which possessed a race consciousness far more pronounced than that of any other in American history.[62]

Eugenicists' racial theory carried still another appeal. Until the start of World War I, it was plausible within the existing framework of scientific knowledge. Though research of the war years, as mentioned before, showed many of eugenicists' claims to be in error, until the mid-1920's no geneticist of note and only Franz Boas of the leading anthropologists publicly disputed them. Since the turn of the century eugenicists' racial views had even received some important endorsements. A very popular President, Theodore Roosevelt, had spoken alarmingly of "race suicide," of the "differential birth rate," of the "Yellow Peril," and had encouraged "native Americans" to have more children. In 1910 the Dillingham Commission, a federal commission which had been established in 1907 to study immigration to the United States, released its widely publicized report which concluded that immigrants from Mediterranean regions were biologically inferior to other immigrants, thereby giving an unofficial government sanction to racist propaganda against southern and eastern Europeans. After the cease-fire, when the wartime hostility toward Germans came to be transferred to virtually all foreign elements, such ideas found a very wide acceptance among the general public. By that time numerous popular magazines and newspapers had begun to disseminate the Nordic theory, and the public credulously heeded the message.

Though almost all eugenicists espoused the theory of Nordic superiority, one group was much more emotionally committed to this position than the rest. Members of this group entertained far deeper prejudices against immigrants than most other eugenicists, and their personality patterns fit the definition of "racist" given earlier. Madison Grant was the prototype; but this group included other leading eugenicists such as Lothrop Stoddard, a historian, and Ellsworth Huntington, a geographer, both of whom wrote "racial histories" patterned after Grant's book; Harry

61. Baltzell, *Protestant Establishment*, p. 113.
62. The hereditary societies served other purposes besides that of easing the insecurities of a troubled patrician class. In particular, almost all these societies loudly and publicly praised the virtues of *patriotism*. Insofar as they did this at a time when the United States was undergoing unprecedented social unrest as well as the birth pains of industrialization and urbanization, these societies undoubtedly provided the country a stabilizing influence.

H. Laughlin, Superintendent of the Eugenics Record Office; Henry F. Osborn, the noted paleontologist of the American Museum of Natural History; and Prescott Hall and Robert DeC. Ward, the two leading figures of the Immigration Restriction League and leaders of the Committee on Immigration of the American Breeders' Association. In origin they were Easterners (primarily from New York and Boston), Protestant, Anglo-Saxon, and proper old-stock aristocrats. Even though their numbers within the movement were not so large, their influence was great, since most of them had become prominent spokesmen for the movement. They had evinced intense hatred for immigrants long before the general public ever heard of the Nordic race, and they had been obsessed with the idea of restricting immigration for decades. Ward, Hall, Grant, and others had participated zealously in the activities of the Immigration Restriction League since its inception in 1894. Of course, other eugenicists to various degrees also had an emotional commitment to the theory of Nordic superiority, but the group in question represents one extreme of a spectrum. In the eugenics movement they found a useful tool to promote sentiment for selective immigration restriction, and after World War I their "scientific authority" as eugenicists proved of great usefulness to them.

* * *

How may the racist eugenicists be distinguished from those who lacked their rigid, deep, emotional commitment to the theory of Nordic superiority? How may such a judgment of "prejudice" be made from the historical record? Prejudice, after all, is something which few would admit to having, even to themselves. The post-World War I appeal of eugenicists' vision of the inferiority of southern and eastern Europeans was that it seemed to make dislike for those peoples a matter of *science*, not of prejudice or ill-will. If "biology" truly did indicate that non-Nordic races possessed undesirable qualities which did not respond to environmental attempts at improvement, that they could not be assimilated, that they could not appreciate American governmental ideals and institutions, and that they outbred the native, then of course it was foolish and self-destructive to permit such newcomers to enter the United States. Osborn could persuasively argue, "Conservation of that race [Nordic] which has given us the true spirit of Americanism is not a matter either of racial pride or of racial prejudice; it is a matter of love of country, of a true sentiment which is based upon knowledge and the lessons of history rather than upon the sentimentalism which is fostered by ignorance."[63] In urging

63. *Ibid.*, p. ix.

immigration restriction, the majority of citizens, including most eugenicists, undoubtedly believed that such a position was in keeping with the latest results of bona fide biological investigations, however neatly these results may have happened to coincide with their emotions on the matter. The group of racist eugenicists quite naturally joined the rest in claiming that they were merely following the dictates of science. Despite their protestations of innocence, however, there are certain qualities in the racists' writings and letters which suggest strongly that their views on immigration were conditioned mainly by deep prejudice against non-Nordics. No one of these characteristics alone necessarily indicates the presence of prejudice, but taken together they make such a diagnosis exceedingly likely.[64]

First, the writings of these men usually betrayed a peculiar tone, a certain emotional intensity, which was not commonly found in the statements of other eugenicists of the era who spoke on race and immigration. In discussing these matters, the racists employed language replete with unnecessary depreciatory adjectives to describe the non-Nordic newcomers. Grant called immigrants "the great swamp of human misery and degradation";[65] Huntington and Leon F. Whitney, Executive Secretary of the American Eugenics Society, described them as "tares in the wheat" and "genuine human weeds."[66] With little patience for the slow, careful process of scientific investigation, eugenicists urged the immediate implementation of available biological "knowledge," however preliminary, into legislative decree. Their intensity distinguished them from more cautious members of the eugenics movement who might have accepted the notion of Nordic superiority but who approached the subject of race much more dispassionately. Until World War I, for example, Raymond Pearl, a statistical geneticist at Johns Hopkins, supported the eugenics program,

---

64. In selecting criteria to be used as indicators of prejudice, I have followed no one source but have been influenced by several treatments of the subject as well as by personal conversations with psychologists and psychiatrists. Among the best of the published works are Milton Rokeach, *The Open and Closed Mind* (New York: Basic Books, 1960); Gordon W. Allport, *The Nature of Prejudice* (Garden City, New York: Doubleday, 1954); Theodor W. Adorno *et al.*, *The Authoritarian Personality* (New York: Harper and Row, 1950); Roger Brown's chapter discussing the Adorno study in *Social Psychology* (New York: Free Press, 1965); and Morris Ginsberg, "Antisemitism," *Essays in Sociology and Social Philosophy*, vol. 2: *Reason and Unreason in Society* (New York: Macmillan Co., 1957), pp. 196-212. I also found very useful the discussion of prejudice in Arthur C. Nielson III, "The Second Ku Klux Klan: 1915-1928. The Life History of a Social Movement" (Harvard University, unpublished Senior Honors Thesis in Social Studies, 1968), pp. 74-81.

65. Madison Grant to Elihu Root, May 10, 1912, *IRL*.

66. Ellsworth Huntington and Leon F. Whitney, *The Builders of America* (New York: William Morrow and Co., 1927), p. 75.

but he stressed the need for more research and fewer polemics. His descriptions of immigrants lacked the belittling tone of that of a Madison Grant.[67] Davenport also admired the Nordic race, but he realized as well that no one group holds a monopoly on desirable qualities. "The fact is," he wrote, "that no race *per se*, whether Slovak, Ruthenian, Turk or Chinese, is dangerous and none undesirable; but only those individuals whose somatic traits or germinal determiners are, from the standpoint of our social life, bad."[68]

Second, the racist eugenicists expressed a hostile animus toward many "outgroups" simultaneously. Grant spoke disparagingly of everyone except the Nordic. He described the Jews, "whose dwarf stature, peculiar mentality, and ruthless concentration on self-interests are being engrafted upon the stock of the nation";[69] the "ignorant and destitute"[70] Catholics; and Hindus, who "have been for ages in contact with the highest civilizations, but have failed to benefit by such contact, either physically, intellectually, or morally."[71] Negroes, he said, are the Nordic's "willing followers who ask only to obey and to further the ideals and wishes of the master race,"[72] and Indians are so cruel that they can "scarcely be regarded as human beings."[73] Such generalized animosities suggest that prejudice and not fear of an objective threat was operating. So encompassing was the prejudice that the non-Nordic immigrant was regarded as the major cause of *all* of society's ills. Albert E. Wiggam, one of the chief popularizers of Nordic superiority, wrote: "It [heredity and blood] has cost America a large share of its labor troubles, its political chaos, many of its frightful riots and bombings—the doings and undoings of its undesirable citizens. Investigation proves that an enormous proportion of its undesirable citizens are descended from undesirable blood overseas. America's immigration problem is mainly a problem of blood."[74] Immigrants thus provided an explanation for America's troubles, a tangible enemy, an outlet and justification for aggression. The faults inherent in American society were ignored; there was no troubling guilt and self-doubt.

67. See Raymond Pearl, "Breeding Better Men," *World's Work*, 15(1908):9818–24.

68. Davenport, *Heredity in Relation to Eugenics*, p. 222.

69. Grant, *Passing of the Great Race*, p. 14.

70. Madison Grant, *The Conquest of a Continent* (New York: Charles Scribner's Sons, 1933), p. 218.

71. *Ibid.*, p. 53.

72. Grant, *Passing of the Great Race*, p. 78.

73. Grant, *Conquest of a Continent*, p. 157.

74. Albert E. Wiggam, *The Fruit of the Family Tree* (Indianapolis: Bobbs-Merrill Co., 1924), pp. 6–7.

The depiction of group stereotypes further indicates the generalized prejudicial mode of thought. Huntington, for example, wrote a book in which each chapter elaborately described the "character" of one of the several racial types.[75] Care was taken to distinguish the individual from the group so that when necessary individual exceptions could be made to preserve the group image. Osborn thus remarked:

Whatever may be its intellectual, its literary, its artistic or its musical aptitudes, as compared with other races, the Anglo-Saxon branch of the Nordic race is again showing itself to be that upon which the nation must chiefly depend for leadership, for courage, for loyalty, for unity and harmony of action, for self-sacrifice and devotion to an ideal. Not that members of other races are not doing their part, many of them are, but in no other human stock which has come to this country is there displayed the unanimity of heart, mind and action which is now being displayed by the descendants of the blue-eyed, fair-haired peoples of the north of Europe.[76]

With similar intention, one supporter of the Immigration Restriction Act explained, "I am not at all anti-Jewish, for instance. I have many splendid friends who are Jews and I cherish their friendship. But . . . "[77] Such stereotypes were reassuring to the racist, for by identifying an outgroup he automatically became part of an ingroup. The excluded became testimony to the insider's belonging.

Moreover, the racist eugenicists sometimes made preposterous claims to support their predetermined beliefs. In *The Builders of America* (1927), Huntington and Whitney asserted without proof that European nations encouraged and frequently even arranged the migration of shiploads of criminals to America.[78] They gratuitously added that "it was a common practice for illegitimate children to go to America where their shame would no longer hinder them and they could start life anew."[79] In *Racial Realities in Europe* (1924), Stoddard cited a number of famous men and events to illustrate the historical achievements of the Nordic race. After warning the reader that his book "makes no pretension to either completeness or finality,"[80] he proceeded to maintain, without evidence or documentation, that almost all modern achievements have been accomplished

75. Ellsworth Huntington, *The Character of Races* (New York: Charles Scribner's Sons, 1924).
76. Grant, *Passing of the Great Race* (1918 edition), p. xi.
77. Arthur M. Churchill to Albert Johnson, January 12, 1924, *Correspondence*.
78. Huntington and Whitney, *Builders of America*, p. 75.
79. *Ibid.*, p. 75.
80. Lothrop Stoddard, *Racial Realities in Europe* (New York: Charles Scribner's Sons, 1924), Foreword.

by Nordics. "The Nordic's great energy, political ability, and high level of intelligence are vital to Europe's prosperity and progress," he wrote. "Those nations which possess most Nordic blood will tend to be the most progressive as well as the most energetic and politically able."[81] He claimed that the bold New World conquistadores were of Nordic type, as were the geniuses who gave rise to the Renaissance.[82] At a time when anti-German sentiment was still prevalent in America, he pointed out that ever since Germany lost its Nordic element during the Thirty Years' War it has consisted mainly of inferior Alpine stock. Realizing this, it becomes possible to understand such phenomena as "the tactlessness and lack of innate courtesy characteristic of modern Germans"[83] and "the mass-nature of German public opinion, its reliance upon authority, and its submissiveness to strong, masterful minorities."[84] Such allegations were generally not so lurid and scandal-mongering as those of the violently anti-Catholic American Protective Association (which in the 1890's forged anti-American papal encyclicals and published the fraudulent "escaped nun books," such as *Confessions of a Nun* by one Sister Agatha, which purported to expose sexual orgies within convents[85]), but the same psychological processes seem to have been involved.

Their prejudice did not change, but hardened, with time. The case of Grant is illustrative. He expressed the same ideas on race in the 1930's as he had for the preceding twenty years, despite the appearance of new, contradictory evidence.[86] The hard-liners like Grant stood noticeably apart from some of their less closed-minded colleagues who ultimately changed their positions on race. Long a champion of selective immigration restriction, Ross had written a vituperative work on immigration (*The Old*

81. *Ibid.*, p. 21.
82. *Ibid.*, pp. 115, 103-4.
83. *Ibid.*, p. 134.
84. *Ibid.*, p. 136.
85. Gustavus Myers discusses the American Protective Association in *History of Bigotry in the United States* (New York: Random House, 1943), chapters 21 and 22.
86. Compare Grant's *Conquest of a Continent* (1933) with his *Passing of the Great Race* (1916).

In the 1920's and 1930's, eugenicists were not unaware that eminent scientists were challenging their biological views. The well-known biologist and moderate eugenicist, Edwin G. Conklin, even summarized the criticisms of several prominent geneticists in an article which appeared as the leading feature in an issue of the *Eugenical News*. Such hard-liners as Osborn and Wiggam attended the meeting of the Galton Society—a very influential New York City eugenics organization—at which Conklin originally presented his paper. See Edwin G. Conklin, "Some Recent Criticisms of Eugenics," *Eugenical News*, 13(1928):61-65. In this article Conklin agreed with some of the criticisms the geneticists made, though he also felt that a cautious, carefully planned eugenics program could be safely applied.

World in the New, 1914) and through the 1920's had praised the books of racists like Stoddard and Henry Pratt Fairchild.[87] In the 1930's, however, as the spectre of totalitarianism and authoritarianism reared its head, he renounced his belief in what he later called the "Nordic Myth."[88] Similarly, Paul Popenoe, who is known today for his successful work as a marriage and family counselor, at one time had been an avid eugenicist and in the 1930's repeatedly praised Hitler's eugenic sterilization law; nevertheless, he too eventually, though belatedly, altered his opinions.

The eugenicists' attitudes toward immigration in the years following the enactment of the Immigration Restriction Act further indicated their prejudice. After this law had been passed, the immigration question quickly ceased to be a major public issue. Those who had feared immigration objectively could now rest assured since the new act seemed salutary. For many of those who had been prejudiced against the newcomers, it might well have become harder to extract the psychological benefits of prejudice now that a major justification for their bigotry was gone. But the hard-line eugenicists felt their battle had only begun. In 1928 and 1930, Grant and Charles Stewart Davison edited volumes in which they called for increasingly stronger immigration measures.[89] In *Conquest of a Continent* (1933), Grant demanded "first and foremost the *absolute* suspension of all immigration from all countries,"[90] followed by wholesale deportation of aliens and enforcement of a strong eugenics program. Barbara Solomon, in a penetrating study of the men of the Immigration Restriction League, pointed out that "to the end of their lives the New England restrictionists were never satisfied that they had saved America from ethnic deterioration."[91]

The prejudice of these men can be understood. They belonged to a generation of Protestant, native-born Americans of colonial stock which had undergone trying times. In the post-Civil War era of industrialization and urbanization, the native, middle class American became increasingly insecure and alienated. He felt his traditional economic and political leadership slipping away to the industrialist, the trust, the political boss, and

---

87. See Edward A. Ross to C. M. Goethe, June 14, 1920; Ross to J. T. Salter, June 16, 1925; and Ross to Lothrop Stoddard, April 26, 1927; all *EAR*.

88. Ross, *Seventy Years of It*, p. 276 and chapter 27.

89. Madison Grant and Charles Stewart Davison, eds., *The Founders of the Republic on Immigration, Naturalization, and Aliens* (New York: Charles Scribner's Sons, 1928); Grant and Davison, eds., *The Alien in Our Midst* (New York: Galton Publishing Co., 1930).

90. Grant, *Conquest of a Continent*, p. 346.

91. Barbara Miller Solomon, *Ancestors and Immigrants; A Changing New England Tradition* (Cambridge: Harvard University Press, 1956), p. 206.

the factory; and he sensed a similar loss of influence and prestige in the cultural and intellectual spheres. This threat of group displacement is what Richard Hofstadter has called the "status revolution" and, according to his interpretation, represents the dynamic behind the progressive movement.[92] Despite the radical-sounding tone of some of its suggestions for reform, the progressive movement, at heart, represented an effort by the middle class to maintain the values, virtues, and social structure of the old way of life in which that group held a vested position.[93] Nowhere in American society was this threat of group displacement more keenly perceived than among that segment to which belonged the eugenicist-restrictionist—the patrician, native-born families of New England, particularly in the Boston and New York areas.[94] Studies in social psychology have indicated the disastrous consequences that fear of status decline may have for one's psychic equilibrium and have pointed to such fears as an important cause of prejudice.[95] Anti-immigrant sentiment was not uncommon to the progressive mind,[96] but to this group of old-line, aristocratic New Englanders who most acutely felt the threat of group displacement, it became an obsession. The American public was ready to consider selective immigration restriction only following the conclusion of World War I, but these eugenicists had been urging such action for the preceding twenty-five

92. Hofstadter, *The Age of Reform.*
93. The desire of progressives to maintain the old way of life is described by Hofstadter, *ibid.*, and is a major theme of Pickens, *Eugenics and the Progressives.*
94. Solomon, *Ancestors and Immigrants*, interprets the "brahmins" as major victims of the status revolution and examines how their fear of group displacement led them into leadership of the campaign for selective immigration restriction.
95. For some representative studies see Bruno Bettelheim and Morris Janowitz, "Ethnic Tolerance: A Function of Personal and Social Control," *American Journal of Sociology*, 55(1949):137–45; Fred Brown, "A Socio-Psychological Analysis of Race Prejudice," *Journal of Abnormal and Social Psychology*, 27(1933):364–74; and Joseph Greenbaum and Leonard I. Perlin, "Vertical Mobility and Prejudice," in Reinhard Bendix and Seymour M. Lipset, eds., *Class, Status and Power* (Glencoe, Ill: Free Press, 1953), pp. 480–91.
96. Many progressives were hostile toward immigrants because it was the newcomers who overcrowded the city, created the blight of the slum, supported the political machine, and perpetrated so much crime. The fact that many immigrants distrusted the idealistic progressives' efforts at social reform did not lessen the dislike that many reformers had for them. Few progressives at the height of the movement, 1900 to 1914, thought that the solution to the problems of immigration lay in restriction; the majority retained faith in the equalizing power of the American environment and continued to believe that the best approach was to try to "Americanize" the immigrant. Nonetheless, the attitudes of these victims of the status revolution toward immigrants showed considerable disdain and represented the beginnings of what after World War I grew into a general sentiment among many groups.

years. To them the "non-Nordic" immigrant provided a convenient and self-serving explanation for society's—and for their own—ills; a eugenic immigration restriction law seemingly provided a solution to America's social problems without making necessary a change in the structure of society.

The racist argument advanced by eugenicists was a logical one, persuasive once its premises were granted. For a long period in their lives these premises were not challenged. The climate of opinion around World War I, as mentioned earlier, differed greatly from that of today; the upper classes everywhere were conscious of their "superiority," particularly over the colored races. The proof of this theory was what they considered the obvious lesson of history, namely, that the white race had conquered the world and hence must be superior. This was the era when "racial histories" were in vogue—books which would explain a nation's history in terms of its "racial" composition, claiming a nation's status to be determined by the amount of Nordic blood it contained. Civil rights leaders at this time were not trying to prove the intellectual equality of the black man but simply trying to help raise him up and to combat Jim Crow.[97] After the climate had changed and their premises had been shown to be invalid, the hard-line eugenicists failed to revamp their position accordingly, for their racial theories still represented a consistent psychological, if not logical, system. In their thinking these men displayed the properties of the "closed mind."[98] Their racial theories satisfied a psychological need so great that otherwise persuasive contradictory evidence made no impression on them. Prominent authorities did take time to demonstrate to them errors in their thinking. Before a Congressional panel, for instance, Laughlin had to answer the criticisms of the well-known geneticist, Herbert Jennings. Nevertheless, without a conscious sense of being intellectually dishonest, these eugenicists managed to disregard, circumvent, or misinterpret such criticisms. They were not so much sincere and misguided as sincere and incapable of being guided. Their insistence that eugenic theory guide immigration policy for a while gained them many followers; but the times changed, and their inability to change with the times ultimately served to the discredit of the eugenics cause which they attempted to serve.

97. In 1912 the Negro leader Booker T. Washington told a conference of white Southern university presidents: "We are trying to instill into the Negro mind that if education does not make the Negro humble, simple, and of service to the community, then it will not be encouraged." C. Vann Woodward, *The Strange Career of Jim Crow*, 2nd ed. (New York: Oxford University Press, 1966), p. 95.
98. See Rokeach, *Open and Closed Mind*.

3. The Geneticsts

Until around 1915, one of the remarkable features of the American eugenics movement was the high degree of enthusiasm and participation it engendered among experimental geneticists. Early investigators of heredity, men who could understand the implications that Mendel's laws held for man, were pioneers in organizing the movement in the United States. In 1906 the American Breeders' Association (American Genetics Association after 1913) created its influential Committee on Eugenics, an event regarded by many as the formal beginning of the eugenics movement in the United States. In 1910 members of the Station for Experimental Evolution, at the time one of the world's leading genetic research laboratories,[99] organized the Eugenics Record Office, the most important center of eugenic research and propaganda in the country.

Although their percentage among the eugenicists was small, a considerable number of geneticists, attracted by the idea of applying genetic knowledge to human problems, took part in the eugenics movement, often enjoying positions of leadership. During the movement's early years they constituted an important nucleus and helped bring the eugenic cause some measure of scientific respectability. Charles B. Davenport, the leading American eugenicist, was also one of America's prominent biologists and had done important work in the areas of embryology, experimental evolution, and genetics. Harry H. Laughlin, Superintendent of the Eugenics Record Office and editor of the *Eugenical News*, was trained as a geneticist and once taught courses in breeding at North East Missouri State Teachers College. Paul Popenoe, author of one of the most widely read textbooks on eugenics, was a well-known biologist and for years edited the *Journal of Heredity*. Every member of the first editorial board of *Genetics* (1916)—a group which included such respected geneticists as T. H. Morgan, William E. Castle, Edward M. East, Herbert S. Jennings, and Raymond Pearl—participated in or gave support to the eugenics movement at some point during the movement's early history.

What is particularly striking is the enthusiasm of some of these men for the eugenics movement at this time. Until around the start of World War I,

---

99. When genetics started there was little interest in it for its own sake since it was initially developed in order to strengthen the basis of the theory of evolution. William Castle and Charles Davenport had both been evolutionary embryologists before turning to genetics as a result of the rediscovery of Mendel's paper. Most of the other pioneer geneticists also shared their intense interest in evolution. How appropriate that this important early genetics laboratory should have been named the "Station for Experimental Evolution"!

many geneticists felt that the movement's goal of genetically upgrading the human race was urgent as well as technically feasible. Pearl told Davenport, "I doubt if there is any other line of thought or endeavor on which common international discussion and *action* can be so well and so profitably brought about as with eugenics."[100] Edwin G. Conklin, a member of the editorial board of *Genetics*, was of the view: "There is probably no other subject of such vast importance to mankind as the knowledge of and the control over heredity and development. Within recent years the experimental study of heredity and development has led to a new epoch in our knowledge of these subjects, and it does not seem unreasonable to suppose that in time it will produce a better breed of men."[101] The University of Wisconsin's Michael F. Guyer, an important figure in the confirmation of Mendelian theory in the first decade of the century, discussed the subject of eugenics in a popular treatise on genetics, "inasmuch as all available data indicate that the fate of our very civilization hangs on the issue."[102] Davenport felt that because of "the importance of our knowing the laws of inheritance of good and bad strains in the country . . . such [eugenic] studies are perhaps the most important that can be undertaken today."[103]

Considering the traditional aloofness of most scientists from affairs outside the laboratory, it is important to consider what attraction these geneticists could find in a popular social movement. To understand their enthusiasm, it is essential to realize first that these men, like most eugenicists, were greatly influenced by the social and intellectual climate of a day in which naturalism and Herbert Spencer dominated the educated mind in America. Underlying their interest in eugenics was their acceptance of much of the naturalistic thinker's world view.

One particularly influential part of that view was the fear cultivated by Social Darwinistic thought that the quality of American stock was deteriorating. Like many other intellectuals of the late nineteenth and early twentieth centuries, a large number of these geneticists felt that the institutions of education, charity, and medicine, by enabling less "fit" individuals to survive, were interfering with the process of natural selection and therefore endangering the future genetic quality of the American people. Their apprehension was accentuated by the widely held belief in the "differential birth rate," the view, popular since the 1870's, that the

100. Raymond Pearl to Charles B. Davenport, February 24, 1913, *CBD*.

101. Edwin G. Conklin, *Heredity and Environment in the Development of Men* (Princeton: Princeton University Press, 1915), pp. v–vi.

102. Michael F. Guyer, *Being Well-Born* (Indianapolis: Bobbs–Merrill Co., 1916), Preface.

103. Charles B. Davenport to David Starr Jordan, May 24, 1910, *CBD*.

"unfit" procreated far more rapidly than the "fit" and thereby threatened to dilute even more the incidence of "valuable" hereditary characteristics in the population. Since the 1870's their alarm was also intensified by the publication of several studies of "degenerate" families such as the "Jukes" and the "Tribe of Ishmael" which purported to prove that vagrancy, criminality, alcoholism, feeblemindedness, prostitution, pauperism, and other undesirable characteristics are all heredity conditions. To prove their point, these widely publicized investigations presented impressive and frightening family trees in which almost every family member under study lived a notorious and immoral life.[104]

At the turn of the century many geneticists expressed such apprehensions. Perhaps the most outspoken was Davenport, a man resolute in his belief that true human progress could result only through improvements in the germ plasm. As he remarked to Charles W. Eliot, president of Harvard University: "It is my present opinion that advances in medical art, at least, are not working toward the increase in the proportion of men reaching a high level of intellectual or physical capacity. The preservation of 'culls' by modern medicine is possibly, if not probably, pulling down the average faster than the increase in eugenical ideals, leading to an increased production of higher types, can possibly upbuild it."[105] During these years Davenport was not alone among his colleagues in voicing such fears. Albert F. Blakeslee, whose researches on the plant Datura provided insight into several fundamental genetic mechanisms, commented: "Although education has been of service in social evolution, its influence in biologic evolution at the present time is of little service if not of distinct harm to the human race."[106] Conklin wrote, "We cannot avoid the conclusion that although our human stock includes some of the most intellectual, moral, and progressive people in the world, it includes a disproportionately large number of the worst human types."[107] He also warned that "many persons believe that our civilization, like other civilizations of the past, is showing signs of degeneration and decay, that throughout the world the

104. Curiously, though almost all these studies adopted alarmist positions, the first of them, Robert Dugdale's portrayal of the Jukes in 1875, did not. In this study Dugdale carefully tried to balance the influence of heredity and environment, and he even recommended environmental reforms to ameliorate the situation. His words of caution were lost upon most of his popularizers, however, who tended to misinterpret his investigation as a justification of the hereditarian viewpoint. See Haller, *Eugenics*, chapter 2 and 7.

105. Charles B. Davenport to Charles W. Eliot, May 4, 1920, *CBD*.

106. Albert F. Blakeslee, "Corn and Education," *Journal of Heredity*, 8(1917):57.

107. E. G. Conklin (written anonymously), "The Future of America: A Biological Forecast," *Harper's Magazine*, 156(1928):532.

less intelligent and more selfish elements of society are coming to control government, industry, and education, while the best elements are dying out or are losing control."[108] Edward M. East, one of the developers of the multiple gene theory, added, "He [the geneticist] believes . . . that if this remedial prescription [control of reproduction] is not generally accepted and put in practice, man's troubles will speedily multiply as they never have before."[109] Fearing that the hereditary quality of the American people was declining, these geneticists quite naturally began to look for possible solutions to the dilemma.

Principles of biology provided them an answer. Many early geneticists, particularly the younger men, who were reared and educated as evolution was winning its victory, openly expressed their enthusiasm for the naturalistic mind's ideal of searching for biological solutions to social problems. They were confident that a biological analysis would enable many pressing social questions to be solved; a eugenics program was appealing to them because it was the answer suggested by biological science. The Nobel laureate H. J. Muller told Davenport, "I have never been interested in genetics purely as an abstraction, but always because of its fundamental relation to man—his characteristics and means of self-betterment, which constituted the primary source of my interest."[110] East commented, "One is inclined to believe, however, that the unique magnetic attraction of genetics lies in the vision of potential good which it holds for mankind rather than a circumscribed interest in the hereditary mechanisms of the lowly species used as laboratory materials."[111] Davenport wrote, "It was early recognized that this new knowledge [the science of genetics] would have a far-reaching influence upon certain problems of human society—the problems of the unsocial classes, of immigration, of population, of effectiveness, of health and vigor."[112]

So fervent a faith in a biological analysis of social problems is understandable. Like many of the educated middle class of their generation, they had permitted "science" to assume an unprecedently high position in their value system. Trusting no other form of knowledge as they did scientific fact, they developed an unshakable confidence in the capability of biology to serve as a tool of social analysis. Some of them spoke of "biological sociology" as one of the great intellectual advances of the age

108. E. G. Conklin, *The Direction of Human Evolution* (New York: Charles Scribner's Sons, 1921), p. viii.
109. Edward M. East, *Mankind at the Crossroads* (New York: Charles Scribner's Sons, 1924), p. vii.
110. H. J. Muller to C. B. Davenport, August 26, 1918, *CBD*.
111. East, *Mankind at the Crossroads*, p. v.
112. Davenport, *Heredity in Relation to Eugenics*, p. iii.

and predicted that it would be fundamental to all future progress in the study of society. As East put it, "Sociology cannot progress without the genetic point of view."[113] Faith in the social analytical powers of biology became so great in some that they came to regard biology as the secular religion of the day, as an absolute to which they could appeal for guidelines for proper social behavior. For others, the science began to assume the proportions of a God-substitute—an ultimate solution to human problems. Like Galton the century before, some geneticists commonly spoke of the "religion of evolution" and viewed eugenic programs as a moral obligation imposed by this new religion. "The topic [of eugenics] . . . is one in which the bearings of science upon religion are most vital, namely, the origin and destiny of the human race,"[114] Conklin wrote. Pearl said of eugenics: "Its ideals must be introduced into the national conscience like a new religion."[115]

While the nineteenth-century legacy established the context for many geneticists' early interest in the eugenics movement, developments internal to the science of genetics permitted the expression of their interest. These discoveries excited many geneticists, for together they suggested that action could be taken on certain social problems these men considered urgent. Most geneticists readily acknowledged the debt that eugenic theory owed the science of genetics. As Pearl wrote, "We may then say that the experimental study of inheritance in plants and animals is one of the main foundations on which progress in scientific eugenics must rest. Genetics is at once the guide and support of eugenics."[116] What developed was a common hope among many of them that if these findings could explain the problems, then they might ultimately guide the social and medical reforms necessary to correct them.

The first of these crucial findings was the rediscovery of Mendel's laws in 1900. By providing a long-sought explanation for the transmission and distribution of traits determined by single genes from one generation to the next, Mendel's laws permitted geneticists to make predictions about the number and types of offspring to be expected from different types of matings. The laws soon made their impact upon breeding; the imprecise rule that "like produces like" was abandoned, and breeders began basing their methods upon quantifiable biological theory. Pleased with results from breeding, many geneticists quickly became enthusiastic about the

113. Statement by Edward M. East in *What I Think About Eugenics*, p. [1].
114. Conklin, *Direction of Human Evolution*, p. vi.
115. Pearl, "Breeding Better Men," p. 9823.
116. Raymond Pearl, "Genetics and Eugenics," *Journal of Heredity* 5(1914): 388.

possibility of extending Mendel's laws from the breeding of plants and animals to that of better human beings.

A second important development was the emergence of a belief that most and perhaps all traits are determined by single genes acting independently, a belief which was common among geneticists during the first ten years of the century. Acceptance of this principle was important to those geneticists interested in eugenic programs, for it imbued them with confidence in their ability to breed better men. Thinking that a one-to-one correspondence exists between genes and observed traits, they felt certain that Mendel's laws explained the transmission of almost all characteristics and hence that geneticists possessed the knowledge to construct sound and valuable eugenic programs.

The third important development was the rapid acceptance after 1900 of the theory of August Weismann, the famed German embryologist and geneticist. In the late 1880's he had produced experimental evidence that characteristics acquired by an organism from environmental pressures could not be inherited by its descendants. He theorized that all inherited traits of sexually reproducing organisms are produced by "determiners" which reside in the germ plasm and which are sensitive only to those environmental pressures which might influence the germ plasm itself. Weismann's work quite legitimately had the effect of discrediting the prevailing belief among biologists in the inheritance of acquired characteristics, but for a while it was also wrongly applied by many to justify a rigid hereditarianism. Most biologists at first tended to misinterpret Weismann's distinction between germinal and body cells to mean that heredity prevails over environment, even though he had claimed merely that the two are different. They also tended to confuse his conclusion that inherited traits reside in the germ plasm with the statement that all traits are inherited through the germ plasm.[117] Weismann's theory had a profound impact upon the social views of many geneticists because for a while they too tended to view his work as proof of the predominance of heredity over environment. In acknowledging his theory, many of them for a time became pessimistic about the possibility of improving defective individuals through environmental agencies, a pessimism which heightened their interest in eugenics as a method to improve the race.

By suggesting the necessity and feasibility of eugenic reform, these three developments in genetics helped to bring about many early geneticists' involvement with the eugenics movement. At a time when intellec-

117. For a discussion of the reception of Weismann's work see Hamilton Cravens, "American Scientists and the Heredity-Environment Controversy" (University of Iowa, unpublished doctoral dissertation, 1969), pp. 10-13.

tual classes were breaking away from rooted traditions, when established faiths were being critically examined, when religious authority was losing its hold upon educated minds, it is not surprising that genetic discoveries should have had this effect. As Guyer declared, "Certain definite principles of genetic transmission have been disclosed. And since it is becoming more and more apparent that these hold for man as well as for plants and animals in general, we can no longer ignore the social responsibilities which the new facts thrust upon us."[118]

Statements similar to that of Guyer were made by almost every American geneticist of the period interested in eugenics. Blakeslee wrote:

> The comparatively recent discovery that knowledge of the laws of biology may be used in the improvement of cultivated plants and domesticated animals furnished the necessary human interest to bring the subject of genetics into popular appreciation. The realization, further, that man himself is subject to the same laws of life as other animals has merely heightened the interest which has been aroused by the application of scientific knowledge to plant and animal breeding.[119]

East urged that "every one . . . learn the tenets of genetics, for there is a genetic aspect to nearly all the problems of society."[120] Significantly, genetic findings apparently influenced the social views of English geneticists in the same way. In the words of William Bateson:

> So soon as it becomes common knowledge—not philosophical speculation, but a certainty—that liability to a disease, or the power of resisting its attack, addiction to a particular vice, or to superstition, is due to the presence or absence of a specific ingredient, and finally that these characteristics are transmitted to the offspring according to definite, predictable rules, then man's view of his own nature, his conception of justice, in short his whole outlook of the world, must be profoundly changed.[121]

Though non-genetically trained eugenicists also recognized the relevance of work in genetics to the eugenics program, they did not make statements such as these. Developments within genetics weighed far more heavily upon the minds of trained experimentalists since these men had developed a keen perception of individual variation and genetic heterogeneity based upon their own laboratory work. They possessed an awareness

118. Guyer, *Being Well-Born*, Preface.

119. Albert F. Blakeslee, "Corn and Men," *Journal of Heredity*, 5(1914): 511-13.

120. Edward M. East, *Heredity and Human Affairs* (New York: Charles Scribner's Sons, 1927), p. v.

121. William Bateson, *The Method and Scope of Genetics* (Cambridge: Cambridge University Press, 1908), pp. 34-35.

of the significance of subtle genetic differences among organisms of the same species which could be acquired only by first-hand experience. R. A. Brink, a distinguished maize geneticist who received his degree under East at Harvard, recalled an incident in a breeding nursery at the University of Wisconsin which illustrates this point. Brink's group had to be on guard for *Ustilago maydis*, a common smut of maize which produces lesions of various sizes on the leaves, stems, and shoots of the plant. One afternoon a worker in the laboratory discovered that each of fifty plants of a certain strain of maize they were studying possessed this lesion in the same spot on a node of the plant where the lesion normally is not seen. This was an incidental observation which did not affect the experiment, but it did cause other workers in the group to gape astonishedly at the plants and to reflect on the scope and subtlety of hereditary differences.[122] Such incidents, which occurred in genetics laboratories everywhere, provided the investigator an understanding of minute genetic differences which could not be similarly appreciated by the non-investigator. Occurrences such as these impressed the experimentalist with the basic genetic *in*equality of individuals and made him consider the question of eugenic reform in a way impossible for the non-geneticist to understand.

Another indication that genetic findings helped produce many geneticists' interest in the eugenics movement can be found in the non-technical writings of some of these men. Of the fifteen geneticists included in the *Biographical Memoirs* of the National Academy of Sciences who worked prior to 1930, for example, two limited their non-technical writings exclusively to the subject of eugenics, seven others also wrote about more general social or philosophical aspects of science, such as its relation to religion or its place in education, but not a single one wrote all his non-technical articles on general issues—a fact which suggests that their interest in eugenics stemmed not just from a general interest in the relation of science to society but from elements within genetics itself. Each of these nine had published papers prior to 1900, but they began writing on social topics of any sort only after that date—only after modern genetics had been born.

At this time, significantly, there seem to have been no additional factors operating on these geneticists to produce their interest in eugenics. Geographical influences apparently played no role. Geneticists interested in social applications of heredity came primarily from the Atlantic seaboard and Great Lakes states, but by 1920 they were found in every section of the country—a distribution which parallels that of American

122. Conversation with R. A. Brink, September 22, 1970.

geneticists in general at this time. No one conceptual category of genetics seems to have been more effective than others in producing this interest. Among the prominent eugenicists, for example, Charles B. Davenport was a Mendelian experimentalist, Raymond Pearl a biometrician, William E. Castle an animal geneticist, Edward M. East a plant geneticist, and Luther Burbank an experimental breeder. An interest in eugenics apparently did not stem from the influence of any particular institution or teacher. At Johns Hopkins, for instance, certain students of William Keith Brooks, most notably Conklin and Nobel laureate T. H. Morgan, were for a time involved with the eugenics movement; yet others, such as E. B. Wilson, never were. Similarly, of Morgan's best-known students at Columbia—H. J. Muller, A. H. Sturtevant, and Calvin Bridges—Muller and Sturtevant became interested in human applications of genetics, while Bridges did not. No particular religious or family influence seems to have been operating either. Since almost all geneticists of this period were Protestant and descended from early American ancestors, they possessed similar social and religious heritages.

It is difficult to determine precisely how many geneticists became involved with the movement, but it appears that a large percentage of them did so—perhaps as many as half.[123] Forty-two of the one hundred American geneticists who served in 1928 on the General Committee of the International Congress of Genetics had at some time been active in the movement. Not only widely known geneticists were involved with the movement, but lesser known investigators as well, men of the type who received unstarred ratings in Cattell's *American Men of Science*.[124] This can best be seen by examining data from the period after 1915. On the Advisory Council of the American Eugenics Society in 1929, in addition to nine starred geneticists, there were ten non-starred students of heredity. A group of geneticists who wrote statements for a small circular, *What I Think About Eugenics*, consisted almost evenly of non-starred and starred scientists. Between 1914 and 1930, articles appearing in the *Journal of Heredity* on the subjects of immigration, birth control, and eugenics were written largely by non-starred geneticists.

Of course, not every geneticist involved with the eugenics movement held it in equal regard or devoted the same amount of time to it. Many were token members of the movement: they joined eugenic societies but

123. On contemporary standards, the absolute number of geneticists who participated in the movement was small. Since there were far fewer geneticists at that time than today, however, the percentage of them involved with the movement was high.
124. A "starred" rating indicated eminence in one's field. The scientists themselves voted to determine who should be so honored.

did not become active in them. T. H. Morgan's brief participation in the movement was of this sort. For a while he lent his name to the Eugenics Record Office as one of its directors, but his actual service to the office was minimal. Many others, however, considered the movement to be so important that they gladly interrupted their busy laboratory schedules to work in its behalf. Many of them wrote frequent articles on eugenic topics, and a few even campaigned for eugenic legislation. Some, such as Castle, spoke mainly to their fellow scientists in technical journals; while others, like East and Pearl, also appealed to the general public by sometimes writing in non-scientific publications. At this time there were no organizations devoted to social issues comprised solely of geneticists, but the organizations of the eugenics and birth control movements (to which some geneticists also belonged) did provide them institutional outlets to air their views.

Thus, between 1900 and approximately 1915, a high percentage of American geneticists became interested in the eugenics movement. Alarmed by what they considered to be a decline in the hereditary quality of the American people, they joined the movement and supported its program of "positive" and "negative" eugenics in the hope that they could help reverse this trend. As ardent enthusiasts of the movement, these geneticists contributed to its early rapid growth. The roots of their interest in the movement lay deep in the nineteenth century. By imbuing them with an interest in applying scientific tools to problems of man, the naturalistic climate helped initiate a sense of social responsibility among them. In addition, their conservative social assumption that economic and social status indicates genetic fitness, their pessimistic view that the American people were hereditarily degenerating, and their interpretation of eugenics as a "secular religion" were all inherited from nineteenth-century biologists and intellectuals. While this intellectual and social milieu constituted the general cause of their interest in the movement, discoveries within genetics acted as the immediate cause. Genetic findings served as an organizing principle which allowed previous speculation on eugenics to be recouched in quantifiable terminology. Also implicit in these discoveries was the suggestion that a national eugenics program was both feasible and desirable. In acting upon the implications of these findings, the geneticists were motivated by their aforementioned social commitments. This is not to say that they allowed their presuppositions to color their scientific interpretation of the discoveries, which they generally did not, but to suggest that with different social commitments they might have drawn from the discoveries another set of social conclusions from those they in fact did draw.

3

Early Human Genetics: Science and Pseudoscience

1. Human Genetics, 1900–1930

After 1900, biologists started investigating inheritance in man as well as in lower organisms.[1] Research in human heredity began at a tumultuous time in genetics; until 1915 the science was torn by the feud between the "Mendelians" and the "biometricians." The Mendelians, as the term suggests, accepted the generality of Mendel's laws. They adopted an experimental approach to the problems of inheritance, and they primarily studied so-called "discontinuous traits," that is, characteristics which appear in one or another contrasting forms, like round versus wrinkled peas. The biometricians, on the other hand, did not accept Mendel's laws. They investigated the phenomena of heredity with pen-and-paper statistical techniques, and they focused most of their attention upon so-called "quantitative" or "metrical" characteristics, that is, traits which show continuous variation along a scale of measurement, such as height and intelligence in man. America constituted the stronghold of the Mendelians, though England's William Bateson and R. C. Punnett were also prominent in this faction;[2] biometricians enjoyed their greatest influence in England,

1. There are three general histories of genetics: Elof A. Carlson, *The Gene: A Critical History* (Philadelphia: W. B. Saunders Co., 1966); L. C. Dunn, *A Short History of Genetics* (New York: McGraw-Hill Book Co., 1965); and A. H. Sturtevant, *A History of Genetics* (New York: Harper and Row, 1965). Dunn provides the most thorough discussion of work in human genetics and related areas. A brief historical sketch of human genetics is also found in the first chapter of Victor A. McKusick, *Human Genetics*, 2nd ed. (Englewood Cliffs, N. J.: Prentice-Hall, 1969).

2. Lionel Penrose, who knew Bateson, recalls that Bateson was so totally un-mathematical that in connection with gene frequencies he had difficulty distinguishing $2x$ from x^2. His god was Mendel, and he was horrified by the idea that genetic problems could be solved with mathematics. Ironically, Mendel himself was a good mathematician. After graduating from the University of Vienna, he taught physics for

45

where they were led by Francis Galton, Karl Pearson, and W. F. R. Weldon. Throughout these years, research in human genetics in England and America, where the subject was most ambitiously pursued, tended to follow each country's respective national style of study. The majority of early English workers in human genetics usually employed biometrical tools, whereas American investigators at this time commonly followed the Mendelian approach.[3]

The first ten years of the century were a highly productive period for human genetics. Biologists quickly realized that Mendel's laws apply to man as well as other organisms, and within a short time investigators had subjected a host of human traits to genetic study. By the end of the decade, many somatic characteristics in man had been found to obey Mendel's laws. Surprisingly, almost all these traits were pathological conditions, the major exception being the ABO blood system, discovered by Karl Landsteiner in 1900. This fact helps explain why most eugenicists from the start were interested mainly in negative rather than positive eugenics.

That decade also witnessed important advances in the statistical study of genetics and human genetics. The English biometrical school under Galton and Pearson led the way in this work. The biometricians felt that heredity should be studied using large populations rather than individuals, and they devised many of the statistical tools necessary for analyzing data from populations. Though their assumptions about the mechanism of inheritance were incorrect—they did not believe in a particulate theory of heredity based on genes which follow Mendel's laws—they nevertheless developed and applied many important statistical methods, including the coefficients of correlation and regression, the normal or Gaussian curve, the standard error, and goodness of fit by the chi-square criterion. The decade's most important mathematical contribution did not come from the biometricians, however, but from George Hardy, an English mathematician, and Wilhelm Weinberg, a German physician, who in 1908 focused attention on gene equilibrium as the pertinent variable in population genetics. Their work was not immediately appreciated, but it did pave the way for the rapid rise of population genetics which began a decade later.[4]

---

a while! (Conversation with Lionel Penrose, January 28, 1971.) See also the biographical note on Mendel in William Bateson, *Mendel's Principles of Heredity* (Cambridge: Cambridge University Press, 1909), p. 311.

3. By 1915 the Mendelians had emerged victorious in this dispute, for the validity of Mendel's laws had become universally recognized. Quantitative traits studied by biometricians could be understood as the result of many genes, each of which separately behaved as a "Mendelian" gene. Cf. pp. 76–77.

4. To be discussed in Chapters 4 and 7. See also Dunn, *Short History of Genetics*, chapter 12.

The most significant achievement in human genetics of the decade was Archibald Garrod's study of genetic blocks in chains of metabolic reactions. In 1902 the English physician showed that alkaptonuria (a metabolic disorder in which the presence in the urine of a substance called alkapton causes it to turn black upon standing) follows a Mendelian recessive pattern of inheritance, and he recognized that parental consanguinity increases the chance that a child will have this condition. In 1908, after a further study of alkaptonuria and other hereditary disorders, he proposed that certain genetic conditions called "inborn errors of metabolism" are caused by a deficiency in enzymes catalyzing particular metabolic steps. Since these diseases are determined by single genes, his work contained the implication that genes function by producing specific enzymes (the "one-gene—one-enzyme" idea), a concept which later played a central role in the development of the theory of gene action. He also propounded the idea of chemical individuality, the notion that there is biochemical diversity within a species, and he suggested that this concept could help explain the nature of differences between species and of evolution in general. Garrod's work was not understood by his contemporaries—indeed, it received little recognition for over forty years—but it foreshadowed many central ideas in biochemical genetics today.[5]

Despite these important discoveries in human genetics, however, not all was well with the field. Enthusiasm for the subject quickly faded, especially in America. By the 1930's the field was disorganized and struggling for survival. Few original studies in human heredity were being undertaken; training programs for human geneticists were non-existent; positions for investigators were exceedingly scarce; and most medical schools of the day omitted the teaching of even rudimentary genetic principles. By 1940 investigations of human inheritance had reached their nadir. Addressing a symposium in 1958, the eminent human geneticist James V. Neel recounted to his younger colleagues "the parlous state of human genetics a scant 15 or 20 years ago. The change in the intellectual—and financial—climate is truly staggering. I well recall how, at the time I abandoned Drosophila in favor of man as an object of genetic research, it was consid-

---

5. See Garrod, "The Incidence of Alkaptonuria: A Study in Chemical Individuality," *Lancet*, 2 (1902): 1616–20; Garrod, *Inborn Errors of Metabolism*, reprinted with supplement by H. Harris (London: Oxford University Press, 1963); and Barton Childs, "Sir Archibald Garrod's Conception of Chemical Individuality: A Modern Appreciation," *New England Journal of Medicine*, 282(1970):71–77.

George Beadle and Edward Tatum, who shared the 1958 Nobel Prize in Medicine for developing the concept of "one-gene—one-enzyme," performed their investigations without knowledge of Garrod's work. Only afterwards did they learn of his contribution, though since then they have generously praised him on numerous occasions. The question of why Garrod was so long overlooked is an enigma.

ered by many of my friends and associates as a very rash move, on the grounds that not only was it out of the question to do anything significant with human material, but there were just no positions to support the few wishing to work in the field."[6]

The reasons for the decline of human genetics in the 1930's were many and complex. Much of the problem stemmed from the difficulties intrinsic to the use of man as an object of genetic investigation. Human generations are far apart; human traits often defy exact measurement; and human beings are not subject to experimental control or prescribed matings. Definitive research in the field had to await suitable statistical methods which were not yet available, new methods of defining and measuring human physiological and psychological traits, as well as the further development of other branches of genetics in order to supply an adequate background in which to carry out and interpret studies of man. For these reasons the interest of most geneticists had from the start been in the general phenomena of inheritance as observed in lower organisms rather than in their specific expression in man. In addition to these difficulties inherent in the material, the field faced problems of its own creation. By the 1920's human genetics rested upon shaky intellectual foundations, for it had come to be dominated by amateur investigators of low critical standards. The quality of their work was sufficiently poor to tarnish the field's scientific respectability, and they did not improve its image by urging that questionable data be immediately applied to social problems. My intention here is to describe the methods, aims, and character of the discipline in this period.

To appreciate the nature of early human genetics, it is most of all necessary to recognize the field's essential characteristic at this time: its intricate relation with the eugenics movement in all countries and particularly in America. The same persons commonly carried out research in both human genetics and eugenics, and many institutions which served one also served the other. Both geneticists and eugenicists came to regard research in human genetics as research in "pure" eugenics.

An important indication of this relationship is that much of the early research in human genetics was instigated and supported by institutions bearing the name "eugenics." The two most important American organizations for the promotion of research in human heredity were the Committee of Eugenics of the American Breeders' Association and the Eugenics Record Office, both of which were headed by the well-known biologist Charles B. Davenport, whose leadership provided a marked stimulus to investigation in the field. As secretary of the Committee on Eugenics, he

6. James V. Neel, "Opportunities for Research in Human Genetics," *American Journal of Human Genetics*, 11(June, 1959) Part 2:290.

organized subcommittees in 1909 to encourage the pursuit of human genetics in institutions and universities. Among the ten research committees he formed were committees on the heredity of feeblemindedness, insanity, epilepsy, criminality, deaf-mutism, and eye defects. (Also organized at that time was the influential Committee on Immigration, controlled by Robert DeC. Ward and Prescott F. Hall of the Immigration Restriction League.) These committees all boasted prominent figures as members. Davenport established the Eugenics Record Office at Cold Spring Harbor, New York, to serve as a "clearing house" of data on human heredity. There he trained over two hundred enthusiastic young "eugenics field workers" who combed town and country collecting family medical records, and he encouraged private individuals to provide the Office summaries of their family histories. This information was analyzed and filed and served as the raw material for numerous monographs on human inheritance by Davenport and others.[7] In England, the center of investigation of human heredity was the Eugenics Laboratory, directed by Karl Pearson, a statistician and disciple of Francis Galton. Under the Laboratory's auspices, numerous investigators, trained in the statistical methods of Galton and Pearson, studied the inheritance of various human traits.

The entanglement of human genetics and the eugenics movement may be illustrated further. Early in the century, studies of human heredity could be found in many scientific publications in a wide range of fields including genetics, anatomy, physiology, psychology, and anthropology. Medical journals, which sometimes presented material on the inheritance of various diseases, constituted another important outlet. Most papers in medical publications did not have eugenic overtones, though a few did contain pleas to physicians to discourage patients with identifiable genetic defects from having children. Work in human genetics appeared most commonly, however, in publications which devoted considerable attention to eugenics. The most important American journal devoting space to the field was the *Journal of Heredity*, a widely read "popular" of genetics which chiefly presented applications of heredity.[8] It was a wealthy benefactor's

7. Cold Spring Harbor was the site of two related institutions, both founded and directed by Davenport. The Station for Experimental Evolution, organized in 1904 with the financial support of the Carnegie Institution, was a leading laboratory for the study of experimental genetics without particular reference to man. As Davenport became interested in human heredity, he persuaded Mrs. E. H. Harriman to donate money to establish the Eugenics Record Office, which began operation in 1910. In 1918 the two institutions merged to form the Department of Genetics of the Carnegie Institution of Washington.

8. David Fairchild, the founder of the *Journal of Heredity*, was the brother-in-law of the founder of *National Geographic*. Fairchild may have envisioned the *Journal* popularizing heredity in the same way that *National Geographic* popularized geography. (Conversation with Sewall Wright, September 24, 1970.)

interest in the subject of eugenics that brought the money to found the journal,[9] which from its start in 1910 published numerous studies of human heredity and eugenics. Other important channels of communication were the *Bulletins* and *Memoirs* of the Eugenics Record Office.[10] In England, Pearson at the Eugenics Laboratory produced the main human genetics publications: *Biometrika*, the principal journal treating biometric data and methods of analyzing quantitative inheritance; and the *Annals of Eugenics*, now the *Annals of Human Genetics*. He also edited the *Treasury of Human Inheritance*, which summarized all the existing literature on many inherited diseases. The *Treasury* made no attempt to draw conclusions about the mode of inheritance of these diseases, but it was extremely valuable for reference.

A second important feature of early human genetics was that nearly everyone concerned, geneticist and eugenicist alike, regarded investigation in the field as research in "pure" eugenics. Most eugenicists considered their chief investigative task to be that of obtaining from pedigree studies information on the inheritance of various human traits. This concept was reiterated by no less important a figure than Davenport. "Human heredity is the leading branch of eugenical research,"[11] he wrote. *"The great work of the future in eugenics is to determine as accurately as possible the law of heredity of each human trait"* [Davenport's italics].[12]

An indication of the prevalence of this view can be obtained by examining the early texts on human genetics. At this time there were two main English texts on the subject, and both were inspired by their author's concern with eugenics. Davenport's *Heredity in Relation to Eugenics* (1911), considered by many the era's most important treatise on eugenics, devoted over half its pages to a discussion of the inheritance of dozens of human characteristics and came to be recognized as the period's most

9. W. E. Castle to L. C. Dunn, March 20, 1933, *LCD*.
10. The most prestigious American publication of this era in genetics, *Genetics*, founded in 1916, only rarely published work in human genetics, despite the fact that several members of the original editorial board were sympathetic to the field. *Genetics* and *Journal of Heredity* served different purposes. Material published in *Genetics* was experimental and technical and usually contained a new principle or technique. (This is still true today.) Investigation of the routine genetics of various organisms would find no place in that journal. Studies of human inheritance, which were usually designed to apply or to extend principles established in other organisms, quite naturally would only rarely find a place in its pages. (Conversation with Sewall Wright, September 24, 1970.)
11. Charles B. Davenport, "Research in Eugenics," in *Eugenics, Genetics and the Family*. Scientific Papers of the Second International Congress of Eugenics, vol. 1. (Baltimore: Williams and Wilkins Co., 1923), p. 26.
12. Charles B. Davenport, "The Eugenics Programme and Progress Toward Its Achievement," in *Eugenics: Twelve University Lectures* (New York: Dodd, Mead and Co., 1914), p. 7.

important human genetics text as well. R. Ruggles Gates, author of *Heredity and Eugenics* (1923), called *Heredity in Man* and *Human Heredity* in subsequent editions, claimed: "I was impelled to write this book by my interest in Eugenics."[13] He based this work on articles he had written in 1920 for the *Eugenics Review*.[14] Other books also illustrated this feature. Horatio H. Newman opened the section on eugenics in his *Evolution, Genetics, and Eugenics* (1925) with a chapter entitled "The Inheritance of Human Characters, Physical and Mental." In *Genetics and Eugenics* (1916), W. E. Castle included the chapter on "Physical and Mental Inheritance in Man" in the section of the book on eugenics, not in the part of the volume on genetics.

As this view of human genetics as "pure eugenics" took hold, the purpose of the field became confused. A division developed between those workers in human heredity interested in pursuing the subject as a pure science and those desiring to apply their findings immediately to social problems. This constituted the distinction between what writers at the time called "pure" and "applied" eugenics. This rift was deep and never resolved. Always among human geneticists (and among eugenicists as well) there were individuals who deemed legislation and propaganda the immediate imperative, and those who felt that the careful accumulation of knowledge should be the first concern.

In general, those with rigorous medical or biological training tended to be more reluctant to clamor for immediate social applications of genetic theory. Lewellys F. Barker, Professor of Medicine at Johns Hopkins and a member of the Scientific Board of Directors of the Eugenics Record Office, wrote: "True eugenics is, at present, in less danger from its avowed enemies than from those who masquerade as its friends. Hasty and ill-advised legislation is preceding not only the cultivation of public opinion, but also that solid foundation of demonstrable fact which alone would justify lawmaking. Surely much harm may easily result from eugenic zeal without sufficient eugenic knowledge!"[15] Davenport insisted: "For a long time yet our watchword must be *investigation*."[16] "We want, above all, to learn as soon as possible how human characteristics are inherited."[17] Many trained investigators in England also distrusted the euthusiasm of the die-

13. R. Ruggles Gates, *Heredity and Eugenics* (New York: Macmillan Co., 1923), p. vii.

14. *Ibid.*, p. vii.

15. Lewellys F. Barker, "Foreword," in *Eugenics: Twelve University Lectures*, p. xi.

16. Charles B. Davenport, *Heredity in Relation to Eugenics* (New York: Henry Holt and Co., 1911), p. iii.

17. Charles B. Davenport, *Eugenics* (New York: Henry Holt and Co., 1910), pp. 26–27. See also Davenport's letter in the New York *Times*, June 21, 1914, p. 14.

hard eugenicists. Pearson said to Galton, "It seems to me that at present there is so very much spade work to be done, and that we are apt to go astray if we merely discuss without the necessary groundwork of facts."[18] In a lecture to the Eugenics Education Society Bateson told his listeners:

> The eugenist and geneticist will, I am convinced, work most effectively without organic connexion, and though we have much in common we should not be brigaded together. Genetics are not primarily concerned with the betterment of the human race or other applications, but with a problem of pure physiology, and I am a little afraid that the distinctness of our aims may be obscured. Alliances between pure and applied science are as dangerous as those of spiders, in which the fertilizing partner is apt to be absorbed.[19]

Their biological background provided these men a deeper appreciation of the difficulties of investigating human inheritance and a keener awareness of the limitations of available knowledge.

But such individuals were relatively few. Most persons associated with the eugenics movement, including many of the leaders, considered the time already ripe for legislation. The economist Irving Fisher of Yale, for example, stated in his 1921 presidential address to the Eugenics Research Association:

> Needless to say, in any propaganda care must be exercised to prevent the hasty endorsement of unproved methods and theories. But there is ample basis already for a movement the initial purpose of which will not be so much a detailed specific program as a general spread of the idea that eugenics is the hope of the world. Details can wait. Where there is a will there is a way and without a will there is no way at all. While eugenic science is painfully finding the way there is ample work for a propaganda organization to secure the will.[20]

In a presentation to the Second International Congress of Eugenics in 1921, Major Leonard Darwin, son of the evolutionist and an internationally recognized leader of worldwide eugenics, voiced even stronger sentiments. Speaking on the aims and methods of eugenic societies, he predicted: "With every growth in our knowledge of biology and sociology we shall be able safety to enlarge our programme."[21] He considered the

---

18. Karl Pearson to Francis Galton, April 6, 1909, in Karl Pearson, *The Life, Letters and Labours of Francis Galton*, vol. 3-a (London: Cambridge University Press, 1930), p. 379.

19. William Bateson, "Commonsense in Racial Problems," *The Eugenics Review*, 13(1921):325.

20. Irving Fisher, "Impending Problems of Eugenics," *The Scientific Monthly*, 13 (1921):231.

21. Leonard Darwin, "Aims and Methods of Eugenic Societies," in *Eugenics, Genetics and the Family*, p. 17.

need to disseminate eugenic ideas so pressing that "with regard to much of the research work which is so urgently needed, most eugenical societies will indeed have no option but to leave it to others or to leave it undone."[22] He further contented that "the main aim of eugenical societies should now be, whilst leaving geneticists to cultivate their own ground, to formulate a sound eugenic policy based on existing genetic knowledge, and then to promote the translation of every advance in eugenic theory into general practice."[23]

This confusion of purpose between research and application existed not only among different individuals in human genetics but often within the same individual. For example, though David Heron, a colleague of Pearson, pursued the subject mainly as a topic of pure research, his interest in the field apparently arose from a hope that in the future it might be applied to eugenic programs. This hope accounted for his quickness to criticize certain studies of human heredity which he felt were inadequately performed: "The service of man demands the very best that science can produce, and those of us who have the highest hopes for the new science of Eugenics in the future are not a little alarmed by many of the recent contributions to the subject which threaten to place Eugenics . . . entirely outside the pale of true science."[24]

As debate over the purpose of human genetics ensued, the position of Davenport was paradoxical and tragic. As an eminent biologist (in 1912 he was elected to the National Academy of Sciences) and as the acknowledged American leader of both human genetics and eugenics, he was in a position to ensure that eugenic zealots crusading for legislation did not permit their enthusiasm to outdistance what was known about human heredity. Although he made numerous reasonable and cautious statements, he was inconsistent in his pronouncements. He frequently denounced "propaganda," but he interpreted the term to mean something different than most other biologists. He did object to the use of the word "eugenics" by advocates of such endeavors as health and food fads, "fitter family" contests, and baby shows, as well as by proponents of more serious causes like birth control, prohibition, and anti-child-labor legislation.[25] However,

22. *Ibid.*, p. 8.
23. *Ibid.*, p. 8.
24. David Heron, *Mendelism and the Problem of Mental Defect—A Criticism of Recent American Work* (London: University of London, Publication of the Galton Laboratory, *Questions of the Day and Fray*, No. 7, 1913), p. 4.
25. See, for example, Davenport, "The Eugenics Programme and Progress Toward Its Achievement," pp. 1–2; and Davenport, "Presidential Address: The Development of Eugenics," in *A Decade of Progress in Eugenics* (Baltimore: Williams and Wilkins, 1934), p. 19.
In opposing birth control Davenport stood among a minority of eugenicists, and once he even refused a request made by the wife of his friend E. M. East to serve on

he regarded both the eugenic sterilization laws and the Immigration Restriction Act of 1924 as important measures, and occasionally he even campaigned for these bills. He often signed petitions in their behalf, and sometimes he defended them in his public addresses: When other biologists complained about hasty applications of human genetics, they objected primarily to *these* measures, not to those which he did discourage. His attempts to resolve the confusion within human genetics therefore did not succeed.[26]

Like Davenport, Galton too was trapped between a desire to study and a hope to apply human genetics but, unlike his American colleague, he achieved a sensible compromise. His commitment to the ideal of a eugenic society was extraordinarily strong—so strong that it sometimes influenced his interpretation of scientific evidence[27]—but not so strong that it blinded him to the folly of creating such a society hastily or prematurely. He insisted that eugenic programs be implemented only *after* a far firmer base of genetic knowledge had been acquired. "My attitude," he wrote, "which has usually been misrepresented, is to urge serious inquiry into specific matters which still require investigation in the well-justified hope that a material improvement in our British breed is not so Utopian an object as it may seem, but is quite feasible under the conditions just named."[28] The organizer of the Eugenics Laboratory, he became embroiled in its warfare with members of the Eugenics Education Society, a propaganda organization comprised of a miscellaneous group of zealots and cranks. In 1910 the

---

the advisory board of the Birth Control League of Massachusetts. Irving Fisher provided a more typical, if overly optimistic, indication of eugenicists' views toward birth control: "If birth control exercised by individual parents could itself be controlled by a eugenics committee it could undoubtedly become the surest and most supremely important means of improving the human race. We could breed out the unfit and breed in the fit. We could in a few generations, and to some extent even in the life time of us today, conquer degeneracy, dependency and delinquency, and develop a race far surpassing not only our own but the ancient Greeks." Charles B. Davenport to Mrs. E. M. East, November 10, 1916, *CBD*; Fisher, "Impending Problems of Eugenics," p. 223.

26. Two good biographical studies of Davenport are E. Carleton MacDowell, "Charles Benedict Davenport, 1866–1944. A Study of Conflicting Influences," *Bios*, 17(1946):3–50; and Charles E. Rosenberg, "Charles Benedict Davenport and the Beginning of Human Genetics," *Bulletin of the History of Medicine*, 35(1961):266–76. Both studies discuss the sometimes conflicting goals of Davenport's scientific interests and his social views. I have prepared a short biographical sketch of Davenport which will appear in the upcoming supplement volume of the *Dictionary of American Biography*, scheduled for publication in 1972.

27. See Ruth Schwartz Cowan, "Sir Francis Galton and the Study of Heredity in the Nineteenth Century" (Johns Hopkins University, unpublished Doctoral Dissertation, 1969), p. i.

28. Pearson, *Life . . . of Galton*, vol. 3-a, p. 253.

Laboratory published a memoir on the children of alcoholic parents in which the investigators were unable to state that children of alcoholics were less healthy than those of non-alcoholics by the time of school age. This prompted a reply published in the London *Times* by Montague Crackenthorpe, the Chairman of the Society, who termed the conclusion "contrary to general experience" without presenting a single piece of evidence in support of his view. (Not only was Crackenthorpe untrained in the statistical methods employed in the paper, but he later admitted he had not even read the article at the time he wrote the letter!) Despite a conciliatory reply by Galton published in the *Times*, Crackenthorpe and several other officers of the Society continued to attack work published by the Eugenics Laboratory. This placed Galton in a difficult position. As the founder of the Laboratory and the honorary president of the Society, he had hoped the two institutions would be complementary. He felt that by popularizing eugenic ideas the Society could actually be of service to the Laboratory. So great was the antagonism between the two, however, that he almost had to resign from the Society. In the end he did not, but he did write a letter to the *Times* in which he stressed that there was no connection between the two organizations (other than his holding offices in both) and regretted "that much of the criticism of the work of the laboratory is by those who write under a strong bias." The point had been reached where the paths of the Laboratory and the Society diverged.[29]

This internal rift over the direction of human genetics had important consequences for the field. With the domination of the science by men favorable to eugenics, most research tended to involve the collection of pedigrees, for such studies presumably provided the facts of human inheritance necessary for the construction of eugenic breeding programs. Almost all studies of human heredity of the era took that form. Hence, at a time when fundamental mechanisms of heredity were being elucidated, human genetics became almost totally oriented toward particular, not general, problems and began drifting away from the mainstream of genetic science. Davenport maintained: "Mendelian studies in man offer an alluring field for future investigation, not, indeed, for the determination of fudamental laws of genetics but for the application of the laws to that species upon whom all progress in science depends."[30] Thus emerged the feeling, even on the part of workers within the field, that the scope of human genetics was tightly restricted. Even some of those few human

29. *Ibid.*, pp. 403–9.
30. Charles B. Davenport, "Mendelism in Man," in *Proceedings of the Sixth International Congress of Genetics*, vol. 1 (Menasha, Wisconsin: Brooklyn Botanic Garden, 1932), p. 140.

geneticists who did make discoveries of general importance at this time were unaware of the general implications of their work. Wilhelm Weinberg, for instance, made significant contributions to population genetics while studying man, but his attention was focused on human inheritance and he did not emphasize the universal importance of his investigations.[31] The viewpoint of the majority of workers in the field became severely limited.

During this period many geneticists sympathized with the task of human genetics, for they recognized fully that the technical limitations in performing genetic studies on man made progress in the field difficult. Speaking before the First International Eugenics Congress in 1912, Punnett said:

> He [man] must be regarded as unpromising [for genetic study], not only from the small size of his families, the time consumed in their production, and the long period of immaturity, but also because full experimental control is here out of the question. For these reasons man is of interest to the student of genetics, chiefly in so far as he presents problems in heredity which are rarely to be found in other species and can only be studied at present in man himself.[32]

Because of these impediments, most geneticists at the time agreed with the view that research in human genetics was necessarily limited to pedigree studies. They still encouraged such investigations, however, *provided* that they were critically performed by men of scientific standing. Shortly after his above remark, Punnett added:

> Though the direct [experimental] method is hardly feasible in man, much may yet be learnt by collecting accurate pedigrees and comparing them with the standard cases worked out in other animals. *But it must clearly be recognized that the collection of such pedigrees is an arduous undertaking demanding high critical ability, and only to be carried out satisfactorily by those who have been trained in and are alive to the trend of genetic research* [italics mine].[33]

Punnett's words were significant; in effect he had offered early human geneticists acceptance into the scientific community as representatives of a still modest, but legitimate, field. His statement came at a critical time in the development of the discipline. A book such as Davenport's *Heredity in Relation to Eugenics*, which had appeared the year before, could still

31. See Curt Stern, "Wilhelm Weinberg," *Genetics*, 47(1962):5.
32. R. C. Punnett, "Genetics and Eugenics," in *Problems in Eugenics*. Papers Communicated to the First International Eugenics Congress (London: Eugenics Education Society, 1912), p. 137.
33. *Ibid.*, p. 138.

contain in one moderate-sized volume nearly all that was known, or thought to be known, about human inheritance. The subject was young, but it had the potential for growth. Davenport and other leaders in the field had a clear choice. Either they could enforce minimal standards of training and critical exactitude for workers in the field in the hope of "professionalizing" the discipline, or they could neglect to do so and by default invite into human genetics the amateur, fresh with enthusiasm having just read Davenport's book. Unfortunately for human genetics, its leaders took the latter course, a negative act which facilitated entry into the field of dilettantes and persons more committed to the application than to the pursuit of knowledge.

Some early leaders of human genetics not only permitted amateurs to enter the field but actually encouraged it. In 1909, the prologue of a new publication, *The Mendel Journal*, contained the following plea:

> [One object of the journal] is to gather for the Science of Genetics a harvest rich in facts relating to human pedigrees and the inheritance of normal characters as well as of peculiarities. . . . We appeal to all who are acquainted with families in which peculiarities and markedly contrasted normal characters, have run from one generation to another, to send details to the Editor of this Journal. . . . While it is clear that medical men have many unique opportunities for acquiring knowledge of pedigrees of this kind, *it is hoped that contributions from laymen will also be forthcoming* [italics mine].[34]

Davenport frequently praised the field workers and data collectors of the Eugenics Record Office, whom he admitted "know nothing about heredity,"[35] and occasionally he defended them from attack. He once complained that criticism of the field workers "is made by physicians and is part of an assumption of superiority that is so widespread among medical men and is so persistently emphasized by some of them that one is almost led to suspect that it is the result of an understanding in the profession."[36] Some dilettantes made their way into the field despite the best efforts of more critical workers to discourage them. Punnett, in his personal recollections of the early days of genetics, described such a novice, C. C. Hurst, a professional horticulturist and an associate of Bateson: "Now Hurst was a tireless worker and full of ideas, but over-apt to find the 3:1 ratio in

34. "Prologue," *The Mendel Journal*, 1(1909):2–3.

35. Charles B. Davenport and A. J. Rosanoff, *Reply to the Criticism of Recent American Work by Dr. Heron of the Galton Laboratory* (Cold Spring Harbor, N. Y.: Eugenics Record Office, *Bulletin* No. 11, 1914), p. 9.

36. Mrs. A. W. Finlayson, *The Dack Family—A Study in Hereditary Lack of Emotional Control* (Cold Spring Harbor, N. Y.: Eugenics Record Office, *Bulletin* No. 15, 1916), p. iv.

everything he touched. While valuing Hurst's enthusiasm for the cause [Mendelism] Bateson was nevertheless mistrustful of his slickness, for he knew that his critical ability had not been sharpened by passing through the scientific mill."[37]

With such amateur enthusiasts entering the field, much early work in human genetics was sloppy and uncritical and often performed with a built-in bias to find Mendelian patterns of inheritance and to demonstrate the omnipotence of genetic as opposed to environmental influences. Many workers failed to adhere to the same critical standards adopted by investigators in other fields, and frequently conclusions would be drawn from evidence far too scanty to satisfy other biologists. This was especially true for work in human genetics coming from the Eugenics Record Office. In a manual which was required reading for all field workers, Davenport provided his data collectors the following instructions on how to conduct pedigree studies:

The field worker must understand that research, seeking to unravel the laws of inheritance, must work out the genetic nature of each individual studied, hence the necessity of extending the pedigree to all ancestors with collaterals, descendants and consorts of all individuals the make-up of whose germ plasm it is desired to understand. For example, by hypothesis, feeble-mindedness is for the most part a recessive trait and the hypothesis must be tested as follows: The field worker finds a person suffering from feeble-mindedness, a descendant of two normal parents—by hypothesis both of these parents are *simplex* [Davenport's term for heterozygous]; the field worker must understand that each parent will probably have somewhere in his or her ancestry a feeble-minded person and *it is the business of the field worker to make a special search for such person or persons in the pedigree* [italics mine].[38]

As a contemporary critic pointed out, "It is difficult to understand how the field-workers would fail to be 'prejudiced by these [Mendelian] rules' when they are instructed 'to make a special search for the person or persons' who are considered necessary for the support of the Mendelian theory."[39] In investigating the role of heredity in insanity, A. J. Rosanoff and Florence I. Orr invented facts which did not exist:

In the analysis of data it was often necessary in the case of a normal subject to determine whether the case was one of duplex or simplex inheritance. . . . The fact of simplex inheritance we were able to establish in

37. R. C. Punnett, "Early Days of Genetics," *Heredity*, 4(1950):8.
38. Charles B. Davenport, *The Study of Human Heredity* (Cold Spring Harbor, N. Y.: Eugenics Record Office, *Bulletin* No. 2, 1911), p. 9.
39. Heron, *Mendelism*, p. 13.

some cases on the basis of the existence of neuropathic manifestations in the ancestors or collateral relatives of the subject; in other cases this evidence was lacking as our information did not extend to the more remote generations, so that it was necessary to *assume* [italics theirs] the fact of simplex inheritance.[40]

Mrs. A. W. Finlayson, in her study of the Dack Family, a clan of degenerates similar to the Jukes, illustrated the bias toward the role of heredity in development so commonly seen among early workers in human genetics. She concluded that the poor scores of four Dack children on the Binet intelligence test indicated they were feebleminded, despite the facts that "the majority of them [Dacks] have received so meager an education that they can hardly write and only a few ever attended a high school"[41] and that the four children "do not appear on first acquaintance as obviously defective, nor do they seem less intelligent than the average of the Dacks."[42] Such examples of inadequate collection and interpretation of data are numerous.[43]

As preposterous as some of these studies may seem, their main trouble is not that they may not contain some truth but that they were insufficiently critical to establish what actually is true. Consider the attempts to show that the tendency to become angry is a Mendelian dominant. There may be single genes which run in particular families and which do tend to affect temperament in this way. It is difficult to establish this firmly for any family history, however, and even more difficult to determine whether the trait has the same genetic basis in different families. The importance of single major genes in human genetics must not be underrated, and today more Mendelizing traits are known in man than in any other organism;[44] nevertheless, the majority of the early studies did not justify their Mendelian conclusions by sufficient evidence.

40. A. J. Rosanoff and Florence I. Orr, *A Study of Heredity in Insanity in the Light of Mendelian Theory* (Cold Spring Harbor, N. Y.: Eugenics Record Office, *Bulletin* No. 5, 1911), p. 226.

41. Finlayson, *Dack Family*, p. 43.

42. *Ibid.*, p. 43.

43. A notable exception among the graduates of the Eugenics Record Office's field worker program is Dr. Wilhelmine E. Key. She was an inspiring teacher and a woman of sound critical judgment. At Lombard College in Illinois she taught biology to Sewall Wright, the eminent population geneticist, and helped him begin his career in the field. (Conversation with Sewall Wright, September 24, 1970.)

44. The most recent survey shows that in man there are 866 confirmed Mendelian traits and 1010 traits suspected as being Mendelian but not yet proved to be. This compares with approximately 310 genes currently described in the well-studied bacterium *Escherichia coli*. Victor A. McKusick, *Mendelian Inheritance in Man*, 3rd ed. (Baltimore: Johns Hopkins Press, 1971), p. xi; Austin L. Taylor, "Current Linkage Map of *Escherichia coli*," *Bacteriological Reviews*, 34(1970):155.

Unfortunately for early human genetics, Davenport himself often performed uncritical studies of this sort. At the start of his career he did excellent work in zoology, ecology, and biometry, and he fully deserved his election to the National Academy. After 1906 his research interests turned almost exclusively to man, and in pursuing this new area he failed to cast aside the presuppositions of the overzealous Mendelian. He became firmly committed to the notion that almost all traits in man, physical and mental, are inherited in simple Mendelian patterns, and he paid only token tribute to the role of environment in determining a person's makeup. Much of his later research consisted of attempts to demonstrate that such characteristics as wanderlust, musical ability, inventiveness, alcoholism, laziness, truancy, and jealousy are determined by single genes.[45] The fact that a trait did not skip a generation in a family was sufficient proof to him that it was a Mendelian dominant. Perhaps the most famous example of this was his attempt to show that a single dominant gene accounts for the tendency to outbursts of violent temper.[46] Sometimes he twisted data for purposes that were not intellectually legitimate or drew erroneous conclusions from evidence. When investigating temperament, for example, he failed to obtain a close correlation between the observed results and the results expected on the basis of temperament being determined by two unit genes, but he still concluded that his hypothesis was confirmed since "these discrepancies only imply a rather slight error in the classification of the observed cases."[47] He was so convinced that the tendency to become angry is produced by a single dominant gene that in one report he tartly dismissed contrary evidence as owing to "an obvious insufficiency of the record."[48] He often admitted the "complexity" of various traits, but complexity to him meant at most the involvement of two or three genes. In one study he acknowledged that "multiple factors" account for body build and then advanced the hypothesis that the number involved was three.[49] Though he always remained abreast of general developments in biology and frequently commented upon recent work in biochemistry,

45. See, for example, Charles B. Davenport, *The Trait Book* (Cold Spring Harbor, N. Y.: Eugenics Record Office, *Bulletin* No. 6, 1912 and 1919) and Davenport, *Heredity in Relation to Eugenics*.
46. See Charles B. Davenport, *Heredity of Constitutional Mental Disorders* (Cold Spring Harbor, N. Y.: Eugenics Record Office, *Bulletin* No. 20, 1920), p. 366. Davenport's method of study and conclusions with regard to this trait were adopted by other workers. See, for example, Finlayson, *Dack Family*, p. 44.
47. Carnegie Institution of Washington *Yearbook*, 1915, p. 139.
48. *Ibid.*, p. 138.
49. Charles B. Davenport, *Body Build and its Inheritance* (Washington, D. C.: Carnegie Institution of Washington, 1923), pp. 149–52.

endocrinology, mutation theory, and chromosome studies,[50] he never abandoned his simplistic view of human inheritance. Even at the end of his career (he died in 1944) he was still calling the tendency to violent temper a Mendelian dominant[51] and still supporting his theories with by then outdated literature from before the first World War.[52]

Such uncritical work did not pass unchallenged by some of the era's more astute geneticists or human geneticists. The outstanding early criticism of the American work came in 1913 from David Heron of the Eugenics Laboratory in London, who focused his attention on Mendelian studies of mental defects. He argued "that the material has been collected in an unsatisfactory manner, that the data have been tabled in a most slipshod fashion, and that the Mendelian conclusions drawn have no justification whatever."[53] He charged, "The authors have in our opinion done a disservice to knowledge, struck a blow at careful Mendelian research, and committed a serious offence against the infant science of Eugenics."[54] Work coming from the Eugenics Record Office received the brunt of his blows.[55] Heron's position was weakened, however, because of his allegiance to the English school of biometry at the time of its warfare with the Mendelians in America. That was unfortunate. A biometrical bias may partly have motivated his attack, judging from the wording of his opening paragraph,[56] but his fundamental point was to encourage Americans working in the field to employ greater caution. This message was lost upon investigators associated with Cold Spring Harbor, who misinterpreted his criticisms as personal strictures prompted mainly by his adherence to biometry. In a public reply to Heron, Rosanoff retorted, "The unfortunate

50. *Ibid.*, pp. 145–46; Charles B. Davenport, Clyde E. Keeler, and Maude Slye, *Medical Genetics and Eugenics* (Philadelphia: Woman's Medical College of Pennsylvania, 1940), pp. 85–86; Davenport, "Mendelism in Man," p. 140; Charles B. Davenport to John H. Gerould, November 17, 1923, *CBD*; Charles B. Davenport to William Bateson, February 9, 1921, *CBD*. Davenport was slow to adopt the chromosome theory of heredity; in his above letter to Bateson he wrote that it "will require a good deal of work yet before it can be adopted generally." As can be seen in his 1932 paper, however, he was quick to predict the existence of clinical entities corresponding to chromosomal aberrations.
51. See Davenport, Keeler, and Slye, *Medical Genetics*, p. 29.
52. See, for example, Davenport's three guest lectures at the Woman's Medical College of Pennsylvania in 1940. His second lecture effectively summarized his 1911 work, *Heredity in Relation to Eugenics*, and the bibliographies for all three lectures showed a disproportionately high number of references from the World War I years or earlier. Davenport, Keeler, and Slye, *Medical Genetics*.
53. Heron, *Mendelism*, p. 61.
54. *Ibid.*, p. 61.
55. *Ibid.*, p. 12.
56. *Ibid.*, p. 1.

position in relation to the scientific world of the English Biometrical school, to which Dr. Heron belongs, may account in some measure for the temper of the attack."[57] Heron's criticisms were ultimately passed over by most investigators.

The curious feature about the early years of human genetics, particularly the first decade, is that work such as that portrayed above occurred alongside studies of lasting value; this period was marked by a curious admixture of good and primarily bad work in the field. In 1916 Davenport produced a paper, still quoted today, in which he showed Huntington's chorea to be a Mendelian dominant trait;[58] he published other investigations which are now in disrepute. This was the period of Garrod and Landsteiner, but it also was the time of Miss Elizabeth Kite and the other zealous eugenic field workers and their biased studies on the Mendelian inheritances of feeblemindedness. To this writer the situation in human genetics at the time was an unusual one. Ordinarily in science most work is non-spectacular but critically performed; however, in this case legitimate investigations were interspersed with work closely akin to pseudoscience. An example of the type of confusion that reigned at the time can be seen in the bibliography to Davenport and Laughlin's *How to Make a Eugenical Family Study*.[59] Together in the same list of references were such classic biological treatises as Edmund B. Wilson's *The Cell in Development and Inheritance*, W. E. Castle's *Heredity*, T. H. Morgan's *Heredity and Sex*, and William Bateson's *Mendel's Principles of Heredity* alongside propagandist statements by amateurs such as Mrs. John Martin's *Is Mankind Advancing?*, Mrs. Frances Gullick Jewett's *The Next Generation*, Lydia R. Commander's *The American Idea*, and M. S. Iseman's *Race Suicide*. As the 1920's opened, therefore, the purpose of research in human genetics was confused and muddled and the scientific structure of the field already shaky. In this perspective, it will perhaps be more understandable how early human genetics became vulnerable to being drawn into the political fray of the day.

57. Davenport and Rosanoff, *Reply to the Criticism*, p. 29.
58. Charles B. Davenport, *Huntington's Chorea in Relation to Heredity and Eugenics* (Cold Spring Harbor, N. Y.: Eugenics Record Office, *Bulletin* No. 17, 1916). This paper first appeared in *American Journal of Insanity*, 63(1916):195, and in preliminary form in *Proceedings of the National Academy of Sciences*, 1(1915):283. One example of a relatively recent writer citing this study is John W. Gowen, "Genetics and Disease Resistance," in L. C. Dunn, ed., *Genetics in the 20th Century* (New York: Macmillan Co., 1951), p. 406.
59. Charles B. Davenport and Harry H. Laughlin, *How to Make a Eugenical Family Study* (Cold Spring Harbor, N. Y.: Eugenics Record Office, *Bulletin* No. 13, 1915).

2. Medicine and Genetics, 1900-1930

As the intellectual status of human genetics deteriorated, the field received little encouragement, support, or interest from medicine. By this time the "scientific era" of medicine had fully begun, and the profession enjoyed more influence and prestige than at any previous moment in its distinguished history. Had medicine embraced human genetics as a branch of medical science early in the century, it might have provided the field the needed impetus to overcome its shortcomings. Unfortunately for human genetics, this did not happen. Instead, for five decades the profession of medicine in general remained ignorant of and uncordial to advances in genetics.

Some physicians in this period, of course, did make important contributions to human genetics. Garrod, Landsteiner, and Weinberg—all medical men—made pioneering discoveries, and other physicians did significant though less spectacular work. Some doctors helped develop the idea that individuals differ in their hereditary susceptibility to disease. They had a special interest in the so-called "constitutional tendencies" to cancer and tuberculosis.[60] Franklin Mall and other early workers in teratology also were alive to the problems of heredity.[61] So were the many physicians who successfully described the inheritance patterns of various genetic diseases, as well as those pathologists, like Leslie Webster and Lloyd Aycock, who became interested in the hereditary aspects of immunology.

Despite these achievements by individual medical scientists, however, the profession in general paid human genetics strikingly little attention. Physicians performed just a small percentage of the total work in the area at this time. Only nine medical references appeared on the ten page reading list for Curt Stern's first human genetics seminar in 1939.[62] In R. Ruggles Gates's *Heredity in Man* (1930) the bibliographies of seven of the eight chapters dealing with topics other than the inheritance of diseases contained almost exclusively non-medical references.[63] (The one exception was the chapter on the blood groups.) Of the twenty-five books in the

60. See George Draper, *Human Constitution; A Consideration of its Relationship to Disease* (Philadelphia: W. B. Saunders Co., 1924).
61. Mall recognized that birth defects may result from both hereditary factors and external influences which act upon the egg after it is fertilized. See Franklin Mall, *A Study of the Causes Underlying the Origin of Human Monsters* (Philadelphia: The Wistar Institute of Anatomy and Biology, 1908).
62. Copy of reading list in possession of author.
63. R. Ruggles Gates, *Heredity in Man* (New York: Macmillan Co., 1930), chapters 1-4, 15-16.

Johns Hopkins Medical Library dealing with human genetics and eugenics published before 1950, only five were written by physicians.[64] Though many genetic studies were conducted on hereditary diseases, a large part of even that work was performed by individuals other than medical doctors and appeared in scientific rather than medical locations. Gates (who himself was not a physician) devoted nine chapters in his book to different categories of genetic disorders. In five of these chapters the references to non-scientific publications outnumbered those to medical publications by as much as five to one, and in the other four chapters the references to non-medical literature consisted of approximately forty per cent of the total.[65]

Many of those physicians who did pursue genetics, moreover, did so as a hobby or curiosity; few persons at this time considered human or clinical genetics to constitute a branch of medical science. Prior to 1940 textbooks ignored the areas of genetics and metabolic diseases.[66] Throughout this period not a single medical college in America offered its students formal, required instruction in genetics. Some schools included a few lectures on Mendel's laws in anatomy or embryology courses, but only in 1933 at Ohio State did Laurence H. Snyder teach the first required course in genetics to medical students in the United States.

Some of the era's few heredity-minded physicians lamented the lack of attention paid to genetics by their colleagues. Lewellys F. Barker of the Johns Hopkins School of Medicine, considered by many at the time the American physician most knowledgeable on heredity, complained: "To the biologists and especially the geneticists of this country, it must be little short of amazing that American clinicians have been so little influenced either in work or in thought by the stupendous advances that have been made in our knowledge of heredity since the turn of the century."[67] He deplored "the apparent apathy of medical men with regard to the problems of inheritance"[68] and "the sluggishness of our clinics as far as efforts to apply the newer knowledge and technique to the solution of the problems of health and disease in man."[69] Experimental geneticists interested in human genetics expressed similar regrets. Samuel J. Holmes, professor

64. Childs, "Garrod's Conception of Chemical Individuality," p. 76.

65. Gates, *Heredity in Man*, chapters 5–8, 10–14.

66. See the table in Childs, "Garrod's Conception of Chemical Individuality," p. 75.

67. Lewellys Barker, "Heredity in the Clinic," *American Journal of the Medical Sciences*, 173(1927):597.

68. *Ibid.*, p. 598.

69. *Ibid.*, p. 598.

of zoology at the University of California, Berkeley, was dismayed that "at present, the average medical practitioner knows little of genetics. Medical students are fortunate if they pick up a rudimentary knowledge of Mendel's law during their premedical course. In the later grind of regular medical instruction they will probably have few opportunities to make good their deficiencies, even if they should appreciate the importance of so doing."[70]

Not only American medicine ignored genetics, but medicine worldwide. While Holmes was criticizing American medical education, England's J. B. S. Haldane was doing the same of medical education in Britain. "Doctors are not in general taught human genetics," he wrote. "A medical student who has attended three lectures on the entire subject of genetics is unusually well informed."[71] For several reasons, however, the irony of medicine's lack of interest in genetics was particularly great in the United States. Since the time of T. H. Morgan, American geneticists had led the way in the field. Many American geneticists had also engaged in the wide dissemination of their knowledge and discoveries, and their findings had been acclaimed over the world. Some of these men had even written solid popular presentations of genetics which sold extensively and were easily understood by any educated reader. Important works of foreign geneticists were available in every large library, and some had been translated into English. These ironies were forcefully pointed out at the time by Barker.[72]

Underlying the profession's cool reception of genetic science were the practical realities within medicine early in the century. At that time physicians were preoccupied with conquering infectious diseases and improving public and private hygiene. In 1900 tuberculosis and pneumonia were the two leading causes of death in America, and influenza and enteritis were rampant. Medical research bearing upon environmental factors of disease was proving successful, and bacteriology, toxicology, and parasitology had emerged as new fields. It was thus a period when the great majority of

70. Samuel J. Holmes, "A German Text Translated," *Journal of Heredity*, 22 (1931):356. Similarly, H. J. Muller in 1933 complained that "genetically trained physicians and psychologists" are "something as yet non-existent in this country." H. J. Muller, "Human Heredity," *Birth Control Review*, 17(1933):20.
71. J. B. S. Haldane, *Heredity and Politics* (New York: W. W. Norton and Co., 1938), p. 106. In 1932 the noted English biologist Lancelot Hogben likewise pointed out that "at present misguided beliefs about heredity are still widely prevalent in the medical profession owing to the fact that the rapid advances of genetic knowledge in the present generation have not yet had sufficient time to infiltrate the curriculum of clinical studies." Lancelot Hogben, *Genetic Principles in Medicine and Social Science* (New York: Alfred A. Knopf, 1932), p. 202.
72. Barker, "Heredity in the Clinic," pp. 597–98.

patients were victims of environmental agents and when medical research and public sanitation measures everywhere focused upon environmental aspects of disease.

This attention to environmental causes of disease was accentuated by the fact that many sufferers of hereditary conditions passed unrecognized. A man who died of tuberculosis at twenty-five would not live to develop Huntington's chorea in middle age. Newborns afflicted with "inborn errors" such as galactosemia (a disorder of carbohydrate metabolism caused by a deficiency of the enzyme galactose-1-phosphate uridyl transferase) usually died of infection, and a high incidence of infant mortality within a family would not necessarily have suggested the existence of a genetic disorder. Only as antibiotics became used and as infant mortality decreased did many "inborn errors" become noticeable.[73] The lack of discernibility of many sufferers of genetic diseases reinforced the popular view that hereditary conditions were rare and constituted only a minimal portion of the physician's practice.

Since medicine is inherently an applied field, a theme of practicality underlies much of medical education. What differentiates medicine from science, after all, is therapeutics, and medical schools have always found an easier time supporting those "basic medical sciences" known to have diagnostic or therapeutic applications. For many years genetic theory seemed abstruse and apparently unrelated to the problems and needs of the overworked clinician. A physician treating a patient with pellagra could care little more for how a genetic unit was defined than he could for the theory of relativity. To what small degree genetics did touch on medical problems of the day, its knowledge was largely negative and non-constructive. It did a physician little good to know that Huntington's chorea was an inherited condition since that information provided no indication for therapy. A few hereditary or congenital conditions, such as harelip and some forms of hernia, could be successfully treated with surgery. Most hereditary conditions could not be surgically treated, however, and the prognosis of "hopeless" was common. What thus developed among many physicians was a fatalistic attitude toward the power of heredity—a fear that modern medicine was powerless to help patients afflicted with genetic diseases. To the dismay of many experimental geneticists interested in the broader implications of their science, this fatalism about heredity which discouraged physicians was the same fatalism as that popularized by many eugenicists during the debates over immigration restriction legislation in the early

73. This point is made by Childs, "Garrod's Conception of Chemical Individuality," p. 76.

1920's: in either case heredity was portrayed as an omnipotent force.[74] While such fatalism was less important than the above reasons as a cause of medicine's uncordiality to genetic science, it did contribute to that situation, and it is important to this study since it illustrates the interplay of emotion and objectivity in scientific progress.

During the first half of the century this attitude was held by many physicians. In 1927 Barker pointed out that one important reason for "the apparent apathy of medical men with regard to the problems of inheritance" was "the mistaken conception that emphasis upon heredity and constitutional makeup are necessarily conducive to pessimism in therapy and to a paralyzing fatalism."[75] In the 1930's and 1940's this fatalism impeded the crusade of Laurence Snyder, Madge Macklin, and William Allan to have genetics added to the medical curriculum (see Chapter 8). In arguing why medical students should be taught genetics, they had to persuade physicians that medicine could contribute to the welfare of patients suffering from genetic defects.[76] Clarence P. Oliver, the well-known human and radiation geneticist, recalls that the medical staff with whom he attended pathology semanars at the University of Minnesota in the 1930's entertained many misconceptions about genetics. For example, he remembers that Dr. E. T. Bell, the director of the seminars, "used to say on occasion that a certain disease under discussion was hereditary and medical science could not do much for the people, 'so give the case to Oliver.' Then I worked to convince them that such fatalism was not necessary if we knew more about human genetics."[77] Snyder, recounting some of his personal experiences as a human geneticist, remarked:

I think a problem that we should sometimes discuss is assuring the general public, physicians and educators that the mere fact of our establishing a genetic background for a condition does not eliminate the hope of therapy or training as a method of modifying that character. I run into it all the time. The lack of cooperation of many groups with geneticists is largely the fear that if we establish a genetic basis, physicians and educators are not going to be able to use therapy or education or psychology or some other means of improving attitudes, education, and disease.[78]

74. See, for example, Herbert S. Jennings, "Heredity and Environment," *Scientific Monthly*, 19(1924):236–37.

75. Barker, "Heredity in the Clinic," p. 598.

76. See, for example, Laurence H. Snyder, *Medical Genetics* (Durham, North Carolina: Duke University Press, 1940), pp. 8–9.

77. Clarence P. Oliver to author, August 4, 1970.

78. "Problems Confronting Human Geneticists: Discussion," *American Journal of Human Genetics*, 6(1954):109. See also Laurence H. Snyder, "Old and New Pathways in Human Genetics," in Dunn, *Genetics in the 20th Century*, pp. 377–78.

While these men may have overestimated the degree to which physicians were smitten with the fear that hereditary conditions were untreatable—after all, doctors did respond immediately to the use of insulin as a treatment of diabetes mellitus and vitamin B-12 as a treatment of pernicious anemia[79]—there can be little question that many were affected by it.

This attitude toward inherited diseases had an important corollary: the view that heredity could play no part in the manifestation of a trait known to be influenced by the environment. This corollary was useful to physicians of the era, for in an age of novel public health measures it justified their great attention to the environmental aspects of disease. It found its greatest application in discussions of infectious conditions. Many physicians tended to reject the notion that individuals differed in their "hereditary susceptibility" to infection, suggesting instead that such diseases could be completely controlled by combatting the germ. In 1932 E. P. Lyon, dean of the University of Minnesota Medical School and a proponent of the idea that genetics should be taught to medical students, lamented a recent White House Conference he had attended in which that view predominated. "Millions of dollars, it seemed, and millions of words were being expended on environment and not a cent nor a word on heredity,"[80] he complained. "Which part of biology does present-day medicine chiefly apply? The environmental side! You can not get around this fact. Look at the medical journals. Almost all the articles approach disease from the environmental side. I do not know much about the practice of medicine, but thinking of treatment I should say, from pills to prayers, it is all from the outside, all environmental—must be so, for the patient has his heredity already established."[81]

---

79. During the three years following the discovery of insulin in late 1921, for example, the number of articles on diabetes in the medical literature increased over three-fold. During that time the number of pages listed in *Index Medicus* (an indication of total research volume) rose less than fifty per cent. (Data courtesy of Dr. Barton Childs.)

80. E. P. Lyon, "Heredity as a Subject in the Medical Curriculum," *Journal of the Association of American Medical Colleges*, 7(1932):299.

81. *Ibid.*, p. 301.

Eugenicists, not surprisingly, also protested medicine's preoccupation with the environment. Davenport complained: "Modern medicine is responsible for the loss of appreciation of the power of heredity. It has had its attention too exclusively focussed on germs and conditions of life. It has neglected the personal element that helps determine the course of every disease. It has begotten a wholly impersonal hygiene whose teachings are false in so far as they are laid down as universally applicable. It has forgotten the fundamental fact that all men are created *bound* by their protoplasmic makeup and *unequal* in their powers and responsibilities." Davenport, *Heredity in Relation to Eugenics*, p. iv.

The irony of fatalism about heredity was that in fact it was a bogus issue; the fears it engendered were unfounded. A few individuals in both biology and medicine attempted to point this out. Barker declared:

The prejudices against studies of heredity and of constitution [in medical schools] because they are supposed to compel pessimistic and fatalistic ideas in clinical medicine is, from what I have just said, entirely unfounded. . . . We are learning how to change human phenotypes artificially to their advantage; that is one of the functions of medical therapy. Witness, the change in a hyperthyreotic phenotype on excision of one lobe of the thyroid, or that in a hypothyreotic phenotype on feeding thyroxin, or that in a diabetic phenotype producible by hypodermic injections of insulin![82]

Lecturing to students at six Midwestern medical schools, William E. Castle, a mammalian geneticist at Harvard's Bussey Institution, warned his listeners:

Let us not ascribe to heredity familial traits which may owe their occurrence to undiscovered factors in the environment. The student of mental traits and human behavior needs to be particularly on his guard in this respect, since he is dealing with secondary or developed characters which may or may not have a basis in heredity. Even the supposed inheritance of a predisposition to cancer should be studied very critically.[83]

T. Wingate Todd, a prominent anatomist and anthropologist, pointed out "the growing success of preventive medicine, which, recognizing these deviations [certain hereditary defects and diatheses], bends its energies toward keeping them below the threshold of expression. . . . Even so definitely heritable a condition as haemophilia need not now have the terrors which it invoked before the fairy touch of endocrine treatment became possible."[84] In 1927 Herbert S. Jennings, a geneticist at Johns Hopkins, foresaw a day when "defects in genes become as open to remedy as defects in nutrition."[85] He predicted that with the future application of chemotherapy to genetic diseases such a large number of patients would be saved that "in time the race thus accumulates a great stock of these defective

82. Barker, "Heredity in the Clinic," p. 602–3.
83. W. E. Castle, "Heredity: The General Problem and Historical Setting," in *Our Present Knowledge of Heredity* (Philadelphia: W. B. Saunders, 1925), pp. 37–38.
84. T. Wingate Todd, "Review of Holmes' *The Eugenic Predicament*," *American Anthropologist*, N.S., 36(1934):301.
Some English geneticists also tried to combat this fear. See, for example, J. B. S. Haldane, *New Paths in Genetics* (New York: Harper and Brothers, 1942), p. 34.
85. Herbert S. Jennings, "Health Progress and Race Progress. Are They Incompatible?" *Journal of Heredity*, 18(1927):272.

genes."[86] In the light of subsequent events, Jennings' words were prophetic; they anticipated the current debate over mankind's "genetic load," the idea that deleterious mutant genes are rapidly accumulating in the population because modern medicine effectively saves those whom selection otherwise would have eliminated. Despite the eminence of those who belittled the notion that inherited conditions cannot be remedied or improved, however, for several decades that attitude maintained its hold. Only after many more advances in diagnosis and therapy did physicians begin to break its shackles. And it was not until after the atomic bomb was dropped on Hiroshima that the question of "genetic load" dramatically emerged as a public issue.

The above discussion should not be construed to suggest that early in the century only a few unorthodox medical scientists pursued genetics. On the contrary, at this time an interest in heredity could be found among many physicians. In most of these cases, however, the expression of their interest took a form which resulted in little lasting gain for human genetics; the majority of these men were exceptions which illustrated the rule that in this period human genetics received little contribution from medicine. At the turn of the century, for example, some physicians expressed an interest in eugenics. Medical societies were well-represented at the First International Congress of Eugenics in 1912, and that meeting devoted an entire section to "eugenics and medicine." Six physicians, including Sir Rickman J. Godlee, President of the Royal College of Surgeons, and Sir William Osler, were vice presidents of the Congress; and seven served as members of the General Committee.[87] Barker and William H. Welch were on the scientific board of directors of the Eugenics Record Office, and medical doctors could usually be found among the officers of other eugenic societies as well. Davenport frequently lectured on eugenics and human genetics before medical societies,[88] and as secretary of the Eugenics Committee of the American Breeders' Association he formed several subcommittees to promote the investigation of various medical conditions.[89] However, this tentative alliance between medicine and eugenics failed to stimulate physicians' interest in human heredity to the degree that some had hoped. It seemed that eugenics attracted many physicians as

86. *Ibid.*, p. 272.
87. In addition, official delegates were sent from such organizations as the American Pediatric Society, the British Medical Association, L'Académie de Médecine, the Royal College of Surgeons, and the Royal Society of Medicine. See *Problems in Eugenics.*
88. For example, see Davenport, *Eugenics.* This was an invited lecture to the American Academy of Medicine at Yale University.
89. *Ibid.*, p. 29.

a social movement rather than as a science. Men like Welch involved with the movement may have done scientific research at one time, but they were also reformers and "scientific influentials," and it was apparently this latter attribute which prompted much of their early interest in the movement. Furthermore, the alliance between medicine and eugenics was short-lived; by the time of the Second International Congress of Eugenics in 1921, the movement had abandoned its attempt to woo physicians. Eugenicists apparently appealed to physicians ineptly; they did not suggest ways that medicine and eugenics could serve each other within the existing framework of medicine but simply criticized physicians for allowing the weak to survive. Agnes Bluhm told the first eugenics congress: "Medicine has, up to the present time, confined its activities almost entirely to single individuals of its own generation. This science has hardly concerned itself at all with the well-being of future generations; on the contrary, it is bringing to these future generations many evils by its protection of those people who are at present physically or mentally unsound."[90] She said of obstetrics: "Only when a different, Eugenic spirit influences Obstetrics, will it become a blessing and not a curse to the race."[91] The role that some eugenicists suggested for doctors was not that of a healer but of a judge trained to decide who should be permitted to reproduce. One eugenicist claimed: "The future physician must largely be an advisory functionary, rather than a dispenser of medicines. And his advice will be solicited not only for the individual and for the present, but for the race and for the future."[92] Such views were bizarre and uncomfortable to most medical doctors. They discouraged physicians' interest in eugenics and helped to reinforce their belief that medicine was powerless to aid victims of hereditary diseases.

Throughout this period, as I mentioned, some heredity-minded physicians studied the inheritance of various diseases, but many of these men also were exceptions that confirmed the rule. Most physicians of the era who wrote on human genetics had not received any formal preparation in genetics in medical school and had not mastered the methodology of either experimental genetics or of statistical and population genetics, which in the 1920's were rising into prominence. Almost all their research consisted of collecting pedigrees, and while some of it was performed critically and represented important additions to the literature, much of it

90. Agnes Bluhm, "Eugenics and Obstetrics," in *Problems in Eugenics*, pp. 387–88.
91. *Ibid.*, p. 395.
92. H. E. Jordan, "The Place of Eugenics in the Medical Curriculum," in *Problems in Eugenics*, p. 398.

suffered from the same inadequacies discussed in the previous section. Perhaps their most common error was to publish pedigrees of families in which many members were affected with a condition but not those of families in which isolated members were afflicted; this statistical bias provided a misleading notion of the transmission of the trait and of the frequency of the gene in the population. Throughout these years geneticists interested in human heredity acknowledged the contributions physicians potentially could make to the genetics of man, but they were critical of most of the work in heredity then being done by medical doctors. Macklin remarked:

> The geneticist is not in a position to gather the data from which the general principles of human genetics are drawn; the physician is the only one who can do that. But he is not trained and hence much of his record gathering is useless for the medical geneticists who would use his data together with those of other physicians for formulating laws. Thus in reporting a case of inherited disease, he may inquire as to whether the parents were related, but if they say no, he does not record that fact.[93]

Investigators who used the *Treasury of Human Inheritance* often complained that some of the pedigrees they studied were incorrect. The *Treasury* depended on the data of medical men who did not always know what questions to ask or what information to record.[94] It was not until the 1940's that this situation began to change.[95]

Thus, despite their early flirtations with the field, neither physicians nor geneticists for over four decades embraced the cause of human genetics. Physicians of the day encountered illnesses resulting mainly from infection and malnutrition and accordingly they directed their attention to

93. Madge T. Macklin, "Heredity and the Physician," *Scientific Monthly*, 52 (1941):66.

94. Conversation with Lionel Penrose, January 28, 1971.

95. On the other hand, geneticists did not claim that they alone could solve the mysteries of the heredity of man. They typically considered both the geneticist's knowledge of methodology and the physician's understanding of human physiology and pathology to be necessary for the effective pursuit of human genetics. Most of them hoped the field might be explored either by genetically trained physicians or by teams of geneticists, physicians, and psychologists. H. J. Muller wrote: "Medical literature of the past three decades has demonstrated conclusively that little in the way of important results in this field [human genetics] can be obtained by amateurs in genetics, while genetic literature in the same period shows how seldom worthwhile results in regard to human characters that are of real importance in themselves can be obtained by geneticists who are amateurs in regard to the specifically human problems concerned." He felt that "such studies [human genetics] demand the use both of the most specialized knowledge and of the most refined techniques known in biology, medicine and the other specifically human sciences." H. J. Muller, "Human Genetics in Russia," *Journal of Heredity*, 26(1935):193, 196.

environmental causes of disease. They regarded hereditary diseases as very rare and genetic science as abstract and theoretical; they did not appreciate ways in which a knowledge of human genetics could be of practical clinical use to them. Geneticists, as observed earlier, were at the time concerned with the definition of the genetic unit, the elucidation of mechanisms of inheritance and transmission, and the genetic theories of natural selection and evolution, not with the manifestations of these theories in specific organisms. They generally felt that technical impediments made man an unsuitable object for genetic research; the precision and rigor of gene mapping and other procedures in lower organisms made studies of human heredity seem loose and inexact. They turned their attention away from man to Drosophila, Neurospora, and finally microbial genetics, where the prospects for discovery seemed much better. But underlying many physicians' lack of interest in human genetics was a paralyzing fatalism toward inherited diseases which even today still lingers in some corners of the medical world. And underlying most geneticists' appraisal of the discipline was a dissatisfaction with the shallowness of much of the research being conducted in the field. Human genetics had failed to establish its scientific standing and had become vulnerable to political misuse.

4

A Decade of Change: 1914–1924

1. Geneticists

By 1915 the eugenics movement had established itself as an integral part of the American social scene. Eugenic proposals were discussed frequently in magazine articles, public lectures, and circular letters to physicians, teachers, social workers, and clergymen. Membership in eugenic organizations increased; books by eugenicists sold widely and went into many editions; and the subject of eugenics appeared often in newspaper editorials, magazine features, and college curricula. An editorial in the *American Breeders' Magazine* correctly noted that eugenic proposals are "being received more readily among the intelligent and thinking part of the population than the pioneer eugenicists in their fondest hopes have allowed themselves to believe possible."[1] As the movement was gaining in popularity and influence, however, a series of developments within genetics challenged its authority. Taken as a whole, these developments showed that the genetic assumptions underlying the movement were not valid. By demonstrating that heredity was more complex than previously had been thought, they indicated that the difficulties in applying genetic theories to man were correspondingly greater.

Between 1900 and 1909 W. L. Johannsen, a Danish botanist and geneticist, conducted a series of experiments on garden beans which effectively distinguished between inherited and noninherited variation. Johannsen isolated genetically pure lines of beans and tested them for degrees of similarity. Among representatives from different lines he discovered a great deal of variation; among individual plants from the same lines he found no inherited variation but did find much fluctuation resulting from chance

1. "Race and Genetics Problems," *American Breeders' Magazine*, 2(1911):230.

environmental influences. He discovered that inherited variations could be small, environmentally produced variations large, and that the two could be distinguished from each other only by the use of breeding tests. To interpret his observations he introduced the terms "genotype," the genetic makeup of the organism, and "phenotype," the observed character produced by the genes with the environment. These investigations, to the dismay of extreme hereditarians, clearly demonstrated the sensitivity of genes to environmental influences; they showed that development is determined not by heredity alone but by the interaction of heredity and environment.[2]

In 1908 G. H. Hardy of England and Wilhelm Weinberg of Germany derived independently what is known today as the Hardy-Weinberg law, the foundation of modern population genetics. This law gave a mathematical treatment of gene equilibrium in human populations.[3] It implied, among other things, that the elimination of a trait from a population is an extraordinarily long and complex process, thereby belying eugenicists' claim that breeding for or against a particular trait is an easy task. While this principle was not generally appreciated or recognized for the first ten years after its initial exposition, it served as the basis of the important work in population genetics which occurred thereafter, and thus it ultimately established the foundation of one of the most convincing scientific repudiations of eugenicists' scientific world view.

Between 1910 and 1913 the American geneticists Edward M. East and Rollins A. Emerson accumulated crucial evidence which disproved the notion that most, if not all, traits are determined by single genes. Studying

2. See W. Johannsen, *Om Arvelighed i Samfund og i rene Linier. Oversigt over det Kgl. danske videnskabernes selskabs forhandlinger #3 forelagt i modet den 6 Feb. 1903*; and Johannsen, *Elemente der Exakten Erblichkeitslehre* (Jena: G. Fischer, 1909).

3. The Hardy-Weinberg equilibrium formula for Mendelian populations may be stated as follows: if in a large population p_1 is the proportion of gene A_1 and p_2 is the proportion of gene A_2, then after one generation of random mating the genotypes will attain and remain at the following frequencies:

Genotype	Frequency
A_1A_2	p_1^2
A_1A_2	$2p_1p_2$
A_2A_2	p_2^2

The original papers are G. H. Hardy, "Mendelian Proportions in a Mixed Population," *Science*, 28(1908):49-50; and W. Weinberg, "Über den Nachweis der Vererbung beim Menschen," *Jahreshefte Verein f. Vaterl. Naturk. in Württemberg*, 64(1908):369-82.

"quantitative" characters in several types of plants, they found more genetic variation to be present in the second generation of offspring than in the first. They explained this result by advancing the "multiple gene theory," the doctrine that "quantitative" traits are determined by the inheritance of multiple pairs of genes.[4] This theory brought the study of quantitative inheritance into experimental genetics and thus helped to resolve the breach between the biometricians and the Mendelians; thereafter the two approaches to genetics proceeded together.[5] (The reconciliation was completed in 1918 by the English statistician and geneticist R. A. Fisher, who demonstrated with an extension of the Hardy-Weinberg law that the genetic properties of "quantitative" traits could be explained in Mendelian terms.[6]) As more and more "metrical" characteristics were discovered, particularly in man, the theory also made possible the realization that Mendel's laws describe the pattern of inheritance of relatively few traits, thereby invalidating one of the major genetic assumptions underlying nearly all eugenic proposals of the period.

In addition to these developments in genetics, an important development in psychology helped to discredit eugenic assumptions about heredity. Until World War I eugenicists had gained much public support by helping spread a myth known as the "menace of the feebleminded."[7] This view held that feeblemindedness is hereditary, determined by a single gene, and rapidly increasing in incidence in the population. Though a fallacy, it engendered widespread alarm. The myth came into being at the turn of the century with the popularization of a group of investigations of "criminal" and "immoral" families (for example, the "Dack Family," the "Kallikak

4. See Edward M. East, "A Mendelian Interpretation of Variation that is Apparently Continuous," *American Naturalist*, 44(1910):65-82; and R. A. Emerson and E. M. East, "The Inheritance of Quantitative Characters in Maize," *Bulletin of the Agricultural Experiment Station of Nebraska*, 1913, 120 pp.

A "metrical" trait (e.g., intelligence) is determined by the cumulative effect of numerous genes acting together. Though the observed trait, which represents the sum of the action of all the genes, follows no simple pattern of inheritance, each of the genes individually segregates in a "Mendelian" fashion.

5. In 1904 Karl Pearson, the vigorous opponent of Mendelism, had himself constructed a bridge between biometrical population genetics and Mendelian experimental genetics, though he did not realize that he had done so. See Sewall Wright, "Genetics and Twentieth Century Darwinism," A Review and Discussion, *American Journal of Human Genetics*, 12(1960):368.

6. See R. A. Fisher, "The Correlation Between Relatives on the Supposition of Mendelian Inheritance," *Royal Society of Edinburgh Transactions*, 52(1918):399-433.

7. For information on the myth of the menace of the feebleminded see Stanley P. Davies, *Social Control of the Mentally Deficient* (New York: Thomas Y. Crowell & Co., 1930); and Mark H. Haller, *Eugenics: Hereditarian Attitudes in American Thought* (New Brunswick, N.J.: Rutgers University Press, 1963), chapters 7 and 8.

Family," and the "Tribe of Ishmael"). These investigations had concluded that hereditary feeblemindedness is responsible for almost all forms of anti-social behavior. (All but one of these studies had been conducted by field workers trained at the Eugenics Record Office.) The myth reached maturity after 1910 with the first American trials of the Binet intelligence test; the results of these trials suggested that large numbers of Americans were feebleminded and that the number was increasing. Ironically, much of the "rise" in feeblemindedness was an artifact of the process of urbanization. Since a higher level of literacy is necessary for independent survival in city life than in a domestic rural economy, the percentage of the population incapable of living outside an institution automatically increased as more and more Americans at the turn of the century moved to the city. Because most persons at the time did not understand that it was an artifact, their alarm over the apparent rise in feeblemindedness was heightened.[8]

This myth was destroyed in 1919 by the release of the results of the intelligence tests the United States Army had given inductees during the war. Of the 1.7 million recruits given the Binet Test, the largest number which had yet taken the same test, forty-seven per cent of the Caucasians and eighty-nine per cent of the Negroes were found by eugenic standards to be feebleminded. Eugenicists tried at first to capitalize on these results. In one of the best-known analyses and popularizations of the army tests, Carl Brigham, a disciple of Madison Grant and a believer in the Nordic myth, attempted to find a statistical relation between race and intelligence; he concluded that the test results supported Grant's thesis that Nordics are brighter than Europeans from southern and eastern sectors of the continent.[9] Such efforts were futile, however. The percentage of individuals obtaining low scores was absurdly high; many successful but poorly educated citizens tested as "feebleminded." The test had made no provision for the different backgrounds of those who took it! Brigham's book elicited a chain of criticisms which, if not sufficient to drown out popular belief in the intellectual superiority of Nordics, at least helped to alleviate the fear that the country was becoming feebleminded.[10]

Though the test results convincingly refuted a major eugenic tenet, most geneticists paid little attention to this development. Many geneticists

8. Conversation with Lancelot Hogben, February 2, 1971.
9. Carl Brigham, *A Study of American Intelligence* (Princeton: Princeton University Press, 1923).
10. See, for example, Kimball T. Young, "Review of *American Intelligence* by C. C. Brigham," *Science*, 57(1923):666–70.

felt that psychological testing was inexact and non-scientific; these men preferred on principle not to cite psychological data for any purpose. Since the aforementioned genetic findings had already convinced them that eugenic tenets were scientifically untenable, they did not require the army tests as further proof. Of the important first-generation geneticists it appears that only Castle ever had occasion to refer to these tests. The tests constituted a blow to the eugenics movement, but they apparently had little influence on the attitudes of most geneticists toward eugenics.

Certain genetic findings, therefore, indicated that earlier views of inheritance needed to be modified, that eugenicists' assumptions about heredity were invalid. As they came to appreciate the implications of these discoveries, most geneticists who had been participating in the eugenics movement began to lose interest in it. Though most of them did not disagree with the movement in principle, they recognized that its legislative suggestions were scientifically unfeasible. In 1914 A. F. Blakeslee, a cytogeneticist then at the Connecticut Agricultural College, discussed how the new genetic findings affected his view of the movement. He declared, despite eugenicists' claims to the contrary, that "in the garden of human life as in the garden of corn, success is the resultant complex of the two factors, environment and heredity."[11] Acknowledging the importance of environment, he felt that society could be improved by noneugenic means, and he warned against intemperately campaigning for legislation. "The enthusiasm, however, with which some would thoughtlessly rush into eugenics and eugenic legislation shows that they may stand in danger of having the new light [discovery of the importance of heredity in development] blind their eyes to the influence of environment as a factor to be considered."[12]

During the war years, as they came to appreciate the complexity of inheritance, other geneticists also began expressing reservations about the feasibility of eugenic programs. In succeeding editions of his *Genetics and Eugenics* (1916, 1919), William E. Castle had taken increasingly conservative positions towards eugenics; in the third edition (1924) he asserted, "We are limited to such eugenic measures that the individual will voluntarily take in the light of present knowledge of heredity. . . . It will do no good, but only harm, to magnify such knowledge unduly or to conceal its present limitation."[13] Two years later he criticized the studies of human heredity coming from the Eugenics Record Office, claiming that the re-

11. Albert F. Blakeslee, "Corn and Men," *Journal of Heredity*, 5(1914):518.
12. *Ibid.*, p. 518.
13. William E. Castle, *Genetics and Eugenics*, 3rd ed. (Cambridge: Harvard University Press, 1924), pp. 374–75.

sults "have been put into too simple and too rigid categories, and a strictly Mendelian statement of results has been adopted oftener than is justified by present knowledge of genetics."[14]

Though the majority of geneticists were adopting an attitude of increasing caution toward the eugenics movement, a small number, the most noted of whom was Davenport, continued to show enthusiasm for the movement. Undaunted by the implications of the work of Johannsen and of East and Emerson, whose studies they knew, these men would not be shaken from their original conviction that long-run improvements in society could result only from improvements in its germ plasm—that "proper matings," as Davenport put it, "are the greatest means of permanently improving the human race—of saving it from imbecility, poverty, disease and immorality."[15] After World War I, when immigration to the United States rose greatly above its war-time level, they also took conservative positions on questions of race and immigration.

With respect to such factors as location, training, and family background, this minority group of geneticists was indistinguishable from the group which was growing unhappy with the movement. Davenport, of early American Protestant ancestry, had been a student of E. L. Mark at Harvard—but so had Jennings and Castle. There was an intellectual distinction between the two groups, however: those who remained enthusiastic about the movement never seemed to appreciate fully the significance of either the multiple gene theory or of the importance of environment in development; neither did they ever recognize the implications that studies in population genetics held for the feasibility of eugenic schemes. Until his death in 1944 Davenport was assigning single gene determinants to such varied and complex traits as stature, temperament, intelligence, and mental illness and was still eulogizing the "powers" of heredity. These were obvious intellectual differences, of course. Further differences between the two groups became apparent in the 1920's and 1930's and will be discussed in Chapter 7.

Throughout World War I the division between the larger body of geneticists, who were turning away from eugenics, and the less cautious, nonscientifically trained eugenicists was not yet complete. Many respected geneticists had not yet wholly accepted the new findings. In 1916 Guyer still felt that heredity was five to ten times more important than environ-

14. William E. Castle, "Eugenics," *Encyclopedia Britannica,* 13th ed. (1926), pp. 1031-32.

15. Charles B. Davenport, *Heredity in Relation to Eugenics* (New York: Henry Holt and Co., 1911), p. 260.

ment and doubted that the multiple gene theory was significant.[16] Nor were scientifically trained geneticists immune to error in their interpretations of work in human genetics. In an otherwise critical address in 1912, Punnett adopted the currently held view that feeblemindedness was a Mendelian recessive trait and declared that it could be bred quickly out of the population—a mistake committed by some prominent geneticists as late as the 1920's.[17] (In 1917 Punnett corrected his position on this matter. In doing so he became the first to calculate the long-term effect of a very simple program of selection.[18]) Furthermore, the problems of the war were immediate and pressing; issues of eugenic significance temporarily lost their importance to many geneticists.[19] Nevertheless, by the end of the war the intellectual split between most geneticists and the majority of eugenicists had become complete. The role of environment in development had been firmly established, as had the multiple gene theory and the Hardy-Weinberg law; few eugenicists but almost all competent geneticists understood these concepts. Accordingly, most geneticists turned their entire attention back to their experiments; they recognized the limitations of eugenic proposals too keenly to remain active participants in the movement. Offered the presidency of the American Eugenics Society in 1926, Jennings declined so that he could devote his time to laboratory research.[20]

16. Michael F. Guyer, *Being Well-Born* (Indianapolis: The Bobbs-Merrill Company, 1916), pp. 295–96, chapter 3.

17. See R. C. Punnett, "Genetics and Eugenics," in *Problems in Eugenics*. Papers Communicated to the First International Eugenics Congress (London: Eugenics Education Society, 1912), p. 137.

18. See R. C. Punnett, "Eliminating Feeblemindedness," *Journal of Heredity*, 8(1917):464. Lancelot Hogben, who had many discussions with J. B. S. Haldane, believes that this paper later had the effect of helping stimulate Haldane's interest in human genetics. (Conversation with Lancelot Hogben, February 2, 1971.)

19. The war itself did create a new eugenic issue, however, the "eugenics of war," whose most noted propagandist was the naturalist and educator David Starr Jordan. Most eugenicists believed that warfare among primitive men had "eugenic" value, since they felt that in hand-to-hand combat the physically superior individuals would triumph. Many of them viewed modern warfare as "dysgenic," however, since they thought that modern technology enabled the weak to destroy the strong, leaving the relatively inferior—physically, at least—to perpetuate the race. As Jordan commented: "The destruction of the strong means the perpetuation of the weak. The loss of the bold, dashing, and courageous means the rule of the cautious, the timid, the time-serving." David Starr Jordan, "The Eugenics of War," *American Breeders' Magazine*, 4(1913):140.

20. Jennings, like many geneticists of the period, felt a conflict between the time-devouring demands of experimental investigation and his desire to popularize the science and to write on its social implications. Although he devoted considerable effort to writing non-technical articles addressed to the lay public, he was besieged by

Despite their growing disillusionment with the eugenics movement, most geneticists at this time did not repudiate it. Their criticisms of the movement lacked a vindictive quality, and they discussed the matter more often in technical publications addressed to their colleagues than in the popular press. Many of them still felt that the movement's goals were sound; their decline in interest resulted mainly from a recognition of the technical difficulties rather than from a disenchantment with the eugenic ideal itself. As late as 1924, East—while harshly criticizing certain eugenic proposals—still declared the movement to represent "a cause fundamentally good";[21] and only three years earlier an array of distinguished geneticists—including such renowned scientists as L. Cuenot, Herbert S. Jennings, C. E. McClung, Calvin B. Bridges, A. F. Blakeslee, George H. Shull, H. J. Muller, R. A. Fisher, C. H. Danforth, A. Franklin Shull, Leo Loeb, and C. C. Little—had presented summaries of their researches to the Second International Congress of Eugenics in New York, hoping that their work would provide the scientific background to appreciate a later section of the congress on human genetics.[22]

Nonetheless, a distinct change in their attitude had occurred. Gone was the unrestrained enthusiasm for eugenics which some had evinced before the outbreak of the war. Replacing it was an attitude of growing caution toward studies of human genetics and their applications to man. In their private correspondence they showed an even greater suspicion of eugenics than they did in their published remarks. Morgan's distaste for the uncritical work on human genetics and eugenics published at the time in the *Journal of Heredity* led him in 1915 to resign from the American Breeders' Association, which produced the journal. He told Davenport his reasons:

For some time I have been entirely out of sympathy with their method of procedure. The pretentious title for one thing, the reckless statements,

more requests for articles and speeches than he could possibly handle. In response to repeated pleas for such articles by G. D. Eaton, editor of *Plaintalk*, Jennings wrote: "I am not primarily a writer, but an experimenter" and "it is mainly only when I *see* a place where there is a great need for setting forth what are the results of investigation that I try to do any writing of a general character—as in 'Prometheus'." Although he campaigned against immigration restriction legislation, he could not devote himself fully to this cause because of a "heavy campaign of work in experimental breeding of lower organisms." H. S. Jennings to G. D. Eaton, October 31, 1927; H. S. Jennings to G. D. Eaton, April 28, 1927; H. S. Jennings to Theodora Jacobs, March 26, 1924; all *HSJ*.

21. Edward M. East, *Mankind at the Crossroads* (New York: Charles Scribner's Sons, 1924), p. vi.

22. See *Eugenics, Genetics, and the Family*. Scientific Papers of the Second International Congress of Eugenics, vol. 1 (Baltimore: Williams and Wilkins Co., 1923).

and the unreliability of a good deal that is said in the Journal, are perhaps sufficient reasons for not wishing to appear as an active member of their proceedings by having one's name appear on the journal. . . . I think it is just as well for some of us to set a better standard, and not appear as participators in the show.[23]

Even Davenport sympathized with Morgan's feelings. "I am afraid the Journal of Heredity does represent American biological science in this field very poorly; indeed so as to make us ashamed at times. . . . I suppose the editor runs short of material and puts in some worthless stuff,"[24] he replied. Several geneticists in 1920 insisted that the International Congress of Genetics scheduled for the next year be held separately from the Eugenics Congress, rebuffing a suggestion by Castle that the two meetings be held jointly.[25] The Eugenics Congress, Morgan told Bateson, would have "little scientific value, in my opinion, and is for social purposes rather than for scientific."[26] As the 1920's opened, therefore, not only was the scientific structure of eugenics faulty, but most geneticists had already come to view the movement with suspicion.

2. Eugenicists

During the war certain changes were occurring within the American eugenics movement. These changes were not specifically related to the details of its legislative program. Despite the evidence from genetics which suggested otherwise, most eugenicists remained certain of the scientific validity of their proposals. Rather, the movement was undergoing certain changes in tone. Taken as a whole these developments brought the movement closer and closer to the political battlefield.

As many geneticists began to lose interest in eugenics, the movement much more than before came to be led by men making rash and pretentious claims about the power of heredity. Some of these men made astonishingly naive assertions. To quote one of the movement's new "prophets," W. E. D. Stokes, a well-known horse breeder and eugenicist: "There is no trouble to breed any kind of man you like, 4 feet men or 7 feet men—or, for instance, all to weigh 60 or 400 pounds, just as we breed horses."[27] Such claims were based upon eugenicists' elementary and un-

23. T. H. Morgan to C. B. Davenport, January 18, 1915, *CBD*.
24. C. B. Davenport to T. H. Morgan, January 21, 1915, *CBD*.
25. T. H. Morgan to William Bateson, April 17, 1920; C. B. Davenport to T. H. Morgan, July 22, 1920; both *CBD*.
26. T. H. Morgan to William Bateson, April 17, 1920, *CBD*.
27. *Eugenical News*, 2(1917):13.

critical understanding of the phenomenon of inheritance; they placed far too much confidence in the influence of the genes, and they were over-eager to find the 3:1 Mendelian ratio in all the traits they examined.

This first transformation in the movement was accompanied by a second one: the rise to prominence within the movement of racists, of whom Madison Grant and Harry Laughlin were the epitomes. Strong in political sentiment, lacking in scientific interest, racially and culturally prejudiced, these men found in the movement a scientific sanctuary. They constituted a vocal, prominent group whose influence exceeded its numbers; after the war they became the movement's major spokesmen. Their propaganda led Pearl to complain, "The literature of eugenics has largely become a min-gled mess of ill-grounded and uncritical sociology, economics, anthropol-ogy, and politics, full of emotional appeals to class and race prejudices, solemnly put forth as science, and unfortunately acknowledged as such by the general public."[28] Though they knew little about genetics, they none-theless addressed the public as if they were authorities on the subject. "The concern of the scientific geneticist in eugenics propaganda," Pearl wrote, "arises from the fact that it is carried out *in his name*. The public is told that the eugenic *pabulum* it is fed is the last and considered word from the science of genetics."[29]

Finally, after the war the distinction between "pure" and "applied" eugenics blurred. Many eugenicists became increasingly interested in pass-ing eugenic legislation. So did many researchers in human genetics, who were voicing their hopes for the immediate social applications of their findings. As Pearl pointed out, Galton's ideal was not being upheld by his alleged followers. "In Galton's case," he wrote, "these two phases [the investigative and the propaganda] were, on the whole, successive in time, with relatively little overlapping. This temporal disparateness has not al-ways been so distinct in the efforts of some of his followers. . . . In recent years the two phases have largely lost their original disparateness and have become almost inextricably confused."[30] Though many geneticists were pointing out that current genetic knowledge promised no quick hereditary improvement of the human race, the new leadership zealously began to prepare the movement for a decade of intensive legislative campaigning.

By the early 1920's, therefore, most geneticists had come to realize that the technical possibilities for eugenic reform were not what they had

28. Raymond Pearl, "The Biology of Superiority," *The American Mercury*, 12(1927):260.
29. *Ibid.*, p. 260.
30. *Ibid.*, pp. 257, 260.

thought them to be ten years earlier. The majority of eugenicists as well as the general public, however, did not share that realization. As America was undergoing its post-war adjustments, the eugenics movement was entering its height of influence and popularity; nearly everyone, except the geneticists, believed that its views were scientifically sound. This proved to be a useful asset to eugenicists as increasingly they became insistent upon passing laws.

5

Political Thrust

As World War I closed, the eugenics movement was preparing for a decade of intensive legislative campaigning. The movement's political activities had begun even before the war, particularly in the area of eugenic sterilization. By 1917, sixteen states had enacted sterilization measures prescribing the compulsory sterilization of certain categories of persons designated as "hereditarily unfit." These early laws were crude, sometimes punitive rather than eugenic in language; and most were eventually repealed, amended, declared unconstitutional, or ignored.[1] After the war eugenicists campaigned for legislation with greater skill, effectiveness, and sense of mission. Much of their attention continued to be directed toward sterilization. By 1931 a total of thirty states had at some time passed sterilization laws; of the twenty-seven bills still operative, all but seven had been enacted since the war. In the 1930's many American eugenicists also applauded the efforts of their German colleagues who had helped formulate the eugenic sterilization measure decreed by Hitler in 1933.

But after the war, though many eugenicists continued to work for sterilization laws, the movement became even more preoccupied with questions of race. The Second International Eugenics Congress, held in New York in 1921, exhibited the changes which were occurring within the movement. The first volume of the proceedings of the congress was largely devoted to the discussion of general genetic problems, but the second volume was dedicated to the discussion of racial issues. "This section of

1. Early sterilization laws were declared unconstitutional on a variety of legal grounds, including cruel and unusual punishment, denial of due process of law, and denial to institutionalized individuals of equal protection by the law.

the Congress resolved itself into a veritable scientific race-congress,"[2] Davenport wrote.

Racial matters interested not only eugenicists, of course, but virtually all Americans. With the country's unique demographic constitution— Indians, Orientals, Negroes, and a diverse population of whites—such matters had always been of paramount concern.[3] Before the Civil War, much discussion had taken place concerning the "superiority" of white men over non-whites. After the Civil War, however, as an increasing percentage of immigrants began to arrive from the non-Anglo-Saxon countries of southern and eastern Europe (the "new" immigrants, in contradistinction to the "old" immigrants of the ante-bellum era who predominantly came from northwest Europe), more and more attention began to be paid to differences within the white race. It was quite common even then to regard the Anglo-Saxon type as superior to the others. A popular nineteenth-century position held that the writings of St. Paul reflected an "Aryan" tone; that Dante had a "Teutonic face"; and that anyone who called Jesus a Jew was either a fool or a liar.[4] Many also believed that personal and racial qualities were fixed by heredity. As early as the English Renaissance, Shakespeare, through Prospero in *The Tempest*, spoke of the primitive man Caliban as "a devil, a born devil, on whose nature/Nurture can never stick." Such ideas appeared frequently in the literature of the late nineteenth century. William Dean Howells' *The Rise and Fall of Silas Lapham* depicted the tension between the "proper" Bostonians and the *nouveau riche* and linked behavior to "blood," not to "breeding." The wide selling novels of Frank Norris, Jack London, and Owen Wister did much to popularize race theories and to glorify the Anglo-Saxon.[5] Racial stereotypes were common not only in American writing but in European thought as well. The chief spokesman of Anglo-Saxon superiority was Rudyard Kipling.

Yet, underneath these seemingly confident assertions of Anglo-Saxon superiority lay a great anxiety. Many "native" Americans spoke disparag-

2. Charles B. Davenport, "Preface," in *Eugenics in Race and State*, Scientific Papers of the Second International Congress of Eugenics, vol. 2 (Baltimore: Williams and Wilkins Co., 1923), p. ix.

3. William Stanton discusses pre-Darwinian racial theories in America in *The Leopard's Spots* (Chicago: University of Chicago Press, 1960). Thomas F. Gossett traces attitudes toward race in the United States from colonial times to the present in *Race: The History of an Idea in America* (Dallas: Southern Methodist University Press, 1963).

4. A. J. Todd, *Theories of Social Progress* (New York: Macmillan Co., 1918), p. 276.

5. The racial notions manifested in the writings of these men are discussed by Gossett, *Race*, chapter 9.

ingly of ethnic minorities, but they also feared that these minorities might become majorities, that they might displace the "old American" stock in numbers and influence. In the decades following the Civil War many Americans developed an intense hostility toward immigrants, and some even began to agitate for the restriction of immigration. During the 1870's and 1890's, particularly violent outbursts of nativism and anti-immigrant hysteria occurred. In the last decade of the century, when anti-Catholicism was rampant and the American Protective Association was at its zenith, the Immigration Restriction League was organized. As early as 1882 the federal government passed the first measure regulating the entry of aliens into the country.[6]

Eugenicists thus did not invent the view of Nordic superiority, but they elaborated and popularized it. In the early 1920's, as their fascination with the Nordic increased, they began to campaign vigorously for selective immigration restriction legislation. Anti-immigrant feeling at that time was unprecedentedly high, and in the hands of eugenicists the view of Nordic superiority became a powerful instrument for mobilizing such sentiment in behalf of restrictive legislation. The Eugenics Committee of the United States of America constituted the most influential lobby in Congress advocating restriction, and prominent eugenicists served as the chief advisors to Albert Johnson, Chairman of the House Committee on Immigration and Naturalization, furnishing him and his committee the biological "justification" of the "inferiority" of southern and eastern Europeans. (The Irish were a special case. Though from northwest Europe, they were considered "inferior" because they were Catholic.) These sentiments were legislated into permanent form by the Immigration Restriction Act of 1924 (the Johnson Act). By requiring that annual immigration from each European nation not exceed two per cent of United States residents listed in the 1890 census who had been born in that country, the bill guaranteed that the proportion of "new immigrants" from southern and eastern Europe would be small. This law was the greatest triumph of the American eugenics movement in national affairs—its one major nation-wide success. For forty-one years the "national origins principle" established in this law served as the basic rule governing the admission of immigrants to the

6. John Higham in *Strangers in the Land; Patterns of American Nativism 1860-1925* (New Brunswick, New Jersey: Rutgers University Press, 1955) ably examines the circumstances which led to the Immigration Restriction Act of 1924. Barbara Solomon in *Ancestors and Immigrants; A Changing New England Tradition* (Cambridge: Harvard University Press, 1956) traces the development of anti-immigration sentiment in New England, focusing especially on the formation and activities of the Immigration Restriction League.

United States. Only with the Celler Act of 1965, which permitted immigrants to be admitted in the order in which they applied (provided that no country send more than 20,000 immigrants in a given year), was the national origins principle abandoned.

Many eugenicists campaigned for other laws as well, including prohibition, birth control, custodial care for "defectives," and various types of marriage regulation.[7] In the majority of these cases, the arguments of eugenicists were at most accessory. For example, many eugenicists supported anti-miscegenation bills, believing that offspring in racially mixed marriages tended to be less fit than either parent. In most states where popular sentiment demanded such measures, however, legislation already had been passed before the appearance of eugenic arguments. With the exception of a few states where eugenicists helped extend and strengthen the laws, eugenics provided only an after-the-fact justification of legislation already extant.[8] Only in the areas of sterilization and immigration restriction were "biological" considerations so obviously relevant and eugenicists so directly influential. In the long run, eugenicists failed in their mission; they never realized their goal of having eugenic sentiments diffuse into the national conscience like a "religion," and during the Great Depression the movement died. Nevertheless, in appraising the impact and significance of the movement, it is essential not to underestimate the importance of its short-term gains.

1. Eugenic Sterilization Laws

The origin of the campaign for eugenic sterilization lay in the interest of late nineteenth-century reformers in alleviating the plight of the afflicted and unfortunate among mankind.[9] At that time emerged a group of

7. For a discussion of the general scope of the political activities of the eugenics movement, see Mark H. Haller, *Eugenics: Hereditarian Attitudes in American Thought* (New Brunswick, N. J.: Rutgers University Press, 1963), particularly chapter 9. For a specific treatment of the role of eugenicists in the prohibition debates, see Bartlett C. Jones, "Prohibition and Eugenics," *Journal of the History of Medicine and Allied Sciences*, 18(1963):158–72.

8. See Haller, *Eugenics*, pp. 158–59.

9. An informative treatment of eugenic sterilization is found, *ibid.*, pp. 21–39, 47–50, 130–41. A less enlightening account is found in Donald K. Pickens, *Eugenics and the Progressives* (Nashville, Tennessee: Vanderbilt University Press, 1968), pp. 86–101. For a discussion of the law in each state, see chapter 2 in Abraham Myerson *et al., Eugenical Sterilization* (New York: Macmillan Co., 1936). For the texts and legislative records of the laws enacted prior to January 1, 1922, see also Harry H. Laughlin, *Eugenical Sterilization in the United States* (Chicago: Municipal Court of Chicago, 1922), chapter 3.

new professions dedicated to improving the lot of the feebleminded, the insane, the alcoholic, the criminal, the pauper, the orphan, the derelict, and the delinquent, while specialized institutions were created for their care. At first the reformers were optimistic about helping such individuals. By the end of the century, however, as more and more of them came to believe that these conditions resulted from deficient heredity, many began to feel that the problems could not be ameliorated or eliminated by environmental procedures. From such persons—criminologists, psychiatrists, physicians, social workers, trained prison and hospital administrators, members of state boards of charities—came the first thoughts of eugenic sterilization as a means of vanquishing the problem of human failure.

During the 1890's the campaign for legislation which would prescribe the sterilization of the "unfit" began in earnest. In 1897 a bill calling for the asexualization of the feebleminded and certain criminals was introduced and discussed in the Michigan state legislature, where it was ultimately defeated. Some enthusiasts proceeded to sterilize even without legal authorization. At the Kansas State Institution for Feebleminded Children, Dr. F. Hoyt Pilcher castrated forty-four boys and fourteen girls before strong public disapproval forced him to stop.[10] Nevertheless, despite these attempts to rally public support, most people at the time did not favor sterilization. The prevailing belief in the inheritance of acquired characteristics made sterilization seem like an unnecessary and extreme measure. Moreover, the only available method was castration, an operation which seemed crude and which had far-reaching aftereffects on the body.

In the years that followed 1900, however, the sterilization campaign acquired considerable momentum, quickly becoming an integral part of the eugenic program. The cause for sterilization had been aided greatly in the late 1890's by the perfection of the operations of vasectomy in men (the cutting and tying of the vas deferens) and salpingectomy in women (the cutting and tying of the fallopian tubes). These surgical procedures were relatively safe and simple, and they did not disturb the body's hormonal balance as did castration. Criminal anthropology, which assumed that hereditary deficiencies were responsible for many of man's physical and mental defects, by 1900 had become a popular fad, convincing many that the conquest of social evils demanded the eradication of unhealthy germ plasm. Weismann's disproof of the inheritance of acquired characteristics engendered much pessimism about the possibilities of environmental reform, and the rediscovery of Mendel's laws seemed to provide steriliza-

10. Leon F. Whitney, *The Case for Sterilization* (New York: Frederick A. Stokes Company, 1934), p. 126.

tion programs with a biological explanation and justification. Indeed, one proponent asserted confidently that sterilization is a procedure "supported by the soundest scientific principles"[11] and devoted a chapter in his book to demonstrating "the relation of Mendelism to sterilization."[12]

With these developments, eugenicists' arguments gained sufficient force to triumph. In 1907 Indiana became the first state to pass a sterilization measure based upon eugenic principles. (A sterilization bill had been passed by the Pennsylvania legislature in 1905 but was vetoed by the governor.) The Indiana law required the compulsory sterilization of inmates of state institutions who were insane, idiotic, imbecilic, feebleminded, or who were convicted rapists or criminals, whenever recommended by a board of experts. Several states soon enacted similar bills, though most of the lawmaking on the issue waited until the 1920's. By 1931, despite the strong opposition of the Roman Catholic Church, which considered the operation an unjustifiable mutilation, thirty states had passed compulsory sterilization measures. Some of these laws applied to a very wide range of "hereditary defectives," including "sexual perverts," "drug fiends," "drunkards," "epileptics," and "diseased and degenerate persons."

The major figure working for sterilization legislation was Harry Laughlin, who in the words of one observer became "a zealot for passing laws."[13] Humorless and dogmatic, he pursued eugenics as if it were a missionary crusade. His interest in sterilization had been fostered by his appointment in 1911 as secretary of the American Breeders' Association's "Committee to Study and to Report on the Best Practical Means for Cutting Off the Defective Germ-Plasm in the American Population," and during the next two decades he assiduously provided information on the subject to sympathetic legislators from many states. Confident of the efficacy of sterilization programs, he felt that a proper goal would be the elimination within two generations of the inheritance lines of "the most worthless one-tenth of our present population" or "the submerged tenth."[14] In 1922, with the publication of his *Eugenical Sterilization in the United States*, he made his most important contribution to the sterilization campaign. This volume, deemed by a contemporary a work of

11. *Ibid.*, p. 130.
12. *Ibid.*, chapter 5.
13. Haller, *Eugenics*, p. 132.
14. Harry H. Laughlin, *Report of the Committee to Study and to Report on the Best Practical Means of Cutting Off the Defective Germ-Plasm in the American Population. II. The Legal, Legislative and Administrative Aspects of Sterilization* (Cold Spring Harbor, N.Y.: Eugenics Record Office *Bulletin* No. 10B, 1914), pp. 132–50.

"profound influence,"[15] was the first book published in America on the topic of sterilization; and throughout the twenties and early thirties it served as a guide for interested lawmakers and citizens. In the work, after reviewing the existing state sterilization bills and proposing a "model eugenical sterilization law" of his own, he defended the scientific validity of such measures. "Eugenical diagnosis," he wrote, "is a biological science, the success of which, in general, depends upon the application of scientific principles, wide experience and common sense."[16] He assured the reader that "while not stated in so many words, the principal end of research and the purpose of books and papers on the subject of human heredity is, in its practical aspect, to enable predictions in hereditary behavior to be made."[17]

The legal and scientific quality of the sterilization laws varied greatly from state to state. Even when the measures were well drawn legally, many opponents still voiced consternation, for they entertained a justified apprehension that the laws might be abused. Some feared that an individual might be forced into an operation against his will, that errors might be made in determining a person's "eugenic value," or that the laws might become an instrument for the persecution of certain groups, particularly the Negroes. These fears were especially troublesome to those who discerned the class biases of many of the supporters of such legislation. Despite eugenicists' claims to the contrary, they observed that sterilizations in America were sometimes conducted with punitive motives. The English biologist J. B. S. Haldane provided several counterexamples to illustrate how class bias occasionally did enter into the enforcement of the sterilization laws in the United States.[18] His colleague Lancelot Hogben pointed out: "There is a strain of haemophilia in the Royal Houses of Europe. No eugenist has publicly proposed sterilization as a remedy for defective kingship."[19] The motives of eugenicists campaigning for sterilization were never entirely above suspicion.

Most geneticists viewed the state sterilization laws unsympathetically. Claiming that the accumulation of knowledge of human heredity should precede legislation, the majority believed that the existing laws were premature. The laws seemed to provoke more public indignation among

15. Whitney, *Case for Sterilization*, p. 128.
16. Laughlin, *Eugenical Sterilization in the United States*, p. 362.
17. *Ibid.*, p. 362.
18. J. B. S. Haldane, *Heredity and Politics* (New York: W. W. Norton and Co., 1938), pp. 102–5.
19. Lancelot Hogben, *Science for the Citizen* (New York: Alfred A. Knopf, 1938), p. 1053.

geneticists in Great Britain than in the United States, perhaps because eugenicists in America had been successful quite early in obtaining such laws whereas eugenicists in England were still trying. Haldane prefaced the American edition of his widely read *Heredity and Politics* (1938) by saying, "I have deliberately chosen examples of what I consider to be abuses of the sterilization laws from the United States rather than from Germany, not from any anti-American sentiment, but because I wished to persuade the British readers that such abuses may occur under a legal system based on English law, and carried out under the criticism of a press somewhat freer than our own."[20]

Despite their scientific weaknesses and their potential for political abuse, the laws for several reasons evoked relatively little concern among geneticists in America. First, some geneticists thought that sterilization in select instances might be effective, particularly sterilization for feeble-mindedness, a condition which some reputable biologists even in the 1920's considered to be a Mendelian recessive characteristic. Moreover, eugenicists themselves were divided over the sterilization issue; many who sympathized with other eugenic proposals agreed with the majority of geneticists that the laws could not be justified by current knowledge. Though prominent eugenicists had helped instigate the measures, they did not have a mandate from the movement. In addition, despite the occasional publicity given to the question of sterilization (Justice Oliver Wendell Holmes's aphorism that "three generations of imbeciles are enough" is still famous), at no time did the topic become a major issue. The laws usually resulted from the persuasion of a few influential individuals, not from widespread sentiment in their favor. Bleecker Van Wagenen, a leading proponent of compulsory sterilization measures, conceded:

While it is true that much public interest has developed in the past few years on the subject of sterilization as a Eugenic measure, and periodical literature discussing it has multiplied, it must be still recognized that there is, as yet, no considerable number of people committed to its propaganda. The laws already enacted have usually been put through by some very small energetic group of enthusiasts, who have had influence in the legislatures. In at least two of the States it was chiefly the work of a physician. In one, of a woman. It is, therefore, easy to understand why little has been actually done. The machinery of administration has to be created. . . . So we must frankly confess that what has sometimes seemed to be, and has been heralded in some corners as a remarkable development in this movement for race betterment, is, as yet, little more than the hobby of a few

20. Haldane, *Heredity and Politics*, pp. 7–8.

groups of people, and does not really indicate the adoption of a settled policy.[21]

Most importantly, however, the laws were generally unenforced. Only in California, where by January of 1935 nearly 10,000 sterilizations had been performed, were there significant efforts to implement the law. Being the home of the Human Betterment Foundation, an organization which campaigned energetically for eugenic sterilization, California was an atypical situation. In other states enforcement was far less vigorous. By January, 1935, less than 20,000 sterilizations had been performed by law in all the United States. Wagenen complained, "Attorneys-general for the several states do not seem anxious to defend suits and appear to encourage delay in putting the laws into operation."[22] Thus, in the last analysis, the sterilization laws in America stood more as a symbol of the potential than of the actual misuse of genetic science. The repercussions were less great than those of events now to be described.

2. The Immigration Restriction Act of 1924

Prior to 1921, except during the years of World War I, European immigration into the United States was virtually unfettered by government regulation. Beginning in 1882, Congress had passed a series of acts which gave it increasing control over European immigration, but none of these acts accomplished much sifting of the incoming masses. In the late nineteenth century many persons started to fear the consequences of unlimited immigration. Foremost among them were three members of the Harvard class of 1889—Prescott F. Hall, Robert DeC. Ward, and Charles Warren—who came to be interested in restricting immigration while they were under the tutelage of some of their college professors and who founded the Immigration Restriction League five years after their graduation.[23] Nevertheless, only after World War I did popular sentiment begin to clamor for the halt of immigration. The result was the Emergency Act of 1921, a temporary measure restricting immigration from any European country to three per cent of the foreign-born of that nationality listed in

21. Bleecker Van Wagenen, "Preliminary Report of the Committee of the Eugenics Section of the American Breeders' Association to Study and to Report on the Best Practical Means for Cutting Off the Defective Germ-Plasm in the Human Population," in *Problems in Eugenics.* Papers Communicated to the First International Eugenics Congress (London: Eugenics Education Society, 1912), p. 477.

22. *Ibid.*, p. 465.

23. See Solomon, *Ancestors and Immigrants*, chapter 5.

the United States census of 1910. In the debates over this act, economic considerations were primary. Most considered restriction to be necessary to ward off incoming Europeans from an already glutted labor market in the industrial centers. Senator William Dillingham, the author of the bill, wrote in his Senate report explaining the proposed legislation, "New problems have been presented as the result of changed conditions in the United States resulting from our peculiar and excessive industrial development and from the changed [economic] conditions which have been caused and accentuated as a result of the World War."[24]

In the discussion of the immigration issue during the next three years, however, racial considerations became foremost. Considerable attention was paid to the fact that most immigrants now came from the countries of southern and eastern Europe. Proponents of restriction began arguing their case on the grounds that the old "American" or "Nordic" type was in danger of being replaced racially by the influx of undesirable, biologically inferior "new" immigrants. These sentiments were incorporated into the Immigration Restriction Act of 1924. The important feature of the new law was not the restriction of immigration to two per cent, but the *selection* among immigrants which was achieved by establishing 1890 as the census year, a date that greatly reduced the relative proportion of "new" immigration. (The laws of 1921 and 1924 pertained only to European immigration. Oriental immigration already had been excluded by previous measures.) One leading supporter, Charles Stewart Davison, honorary chairman of the American Defense Society, declared that the bill would "ensure that the bulk of our immigration from Europe would come from peoples who are closely related to our basic stocks and older immigration, and would thus remove one serious menace to our racial homogeneity."[25]

Until the end of the war, official federal policy embodied an economic, not a biological, view of immigration. Underlying all immigration bills of the period was only one stated principle: the prohibition of the entry of individuals (but not races) deemed undesirable—criminals, polygamists, anarchists, and the feebleminded. Oscar S. Straus, Secretary of Commerce and Labor, wrote in 1907: "Since the period above mentioned [the Civil War] the laws that have been passed upon the subject [of immigration], while in no way hostile to immigration as such, have proceeded upon the general policy of selection, thereby excluding more and more individuals

24. "Emergency Immigration Legislation," *Senate Report No. 789*, 66th Congress, 3rd Session (Washington: Government Printing Office, 1921), p. 10.
25. Charles Stewart Davison to Albert Johnson, December 31, 1923, *Correspondence.*

coming under the designation of 'undesirable'."[26] F. P. Sargent, Commissioner-General of Immigration, stated in 1903: "The great bulk of present immigration proceeds from Italy, Austria, and furthermore, from some of the most undesirable sources of population of those countries. No one would object to the better class of Italians, Austrians, and Russians coming here in large numbers; but the point is that such element does not come."[27] Thus, it was federal policy to "protect" America from foreigners, but the chief threat was considered to be the influx of degenerate persons, not degenerate races.

This principle received an important affirmation from the Dillingham Commission, headed by Senator William Dillingham, which between 1907 and 1910 conducted the major government examination of the immigration question. The conclusions of the commission are worth noting. It urged that "further general legislation concerning the admission of aliens should be based primarily upon economic or business considerations touching the prosperity and economic well being of our people."[28] It recommended the exclusion of aliens "who, by reason of their personal qualities or habits would least readily be assimilated or would make the least desirable citizens."[29] Its chief proposal was "the reading and writing test as the most feasible method of restricting undesirable immigration."[30] (This provision was enacted into law in 1917, over the President's veto.) Though the commission expressed apprehension that the "quality" of the "new" immigration tended to be inferior to that of the "old," it nevertheless endorsed the principle of individual selection and discussed immigration mainly as an economic rather than as a biological issue. The noted eugenicist Irving Fisher, professor of economics at Yale, later complained of what he considered the commission's overemphasis on economics and underemphasis on biology. "The core of the problem of immigration is, however, one of race and eugenics, despite the fact that in the eighteen volumes of the report of the Immigration Commission scarcely any attention is given to this aspect of the immigration problem."[31]

26. *Annual Report, 1907; United States Department of Commerce and Labor* (Washington: Government Printing Office, 1907), p. 7.
27. *Annual Report, 1903; United States Immigration and Naturalization Service* (Washington: Government Printing Office, 1903), p. 70.
28. "Reports of the Immigration Commission," vol. 1 *Senate Document No. 747*, 61st Congress, 2nd Session (Washington: Government Printing Office, 1911), p. 45.
29. *Ibid.*, p. 47.
30. *Ibid.*, p. 48.
31. Irving Fisher, "Impending Problems of Eugenics," *The Scientific Monthly*, 13(1921):226.

Many individuals between 1900 and 1920 urged that the restriction of immigration be considered a biological imperative, but their pleas at that time aroused little public or Congressional response. The best-known entreaty of this sort was Madison Grant's *The Passing of the Great Race* (1916). This work popularized the notion that America had originally been settled by descendants of a genetically pure "Nordic race," biologically superior to the other European "races," which the new immigration now threatened to eradicate from the American blood stream. A highly influential book, it served as *the* major source of inspiration to racial propagandists in the 1920's and helped mold the views of Congress and the public alike. But the major impact of these writings came *after* the war; until then, despite wide circulation in the press, they evoked relatively little fear.

The American mood before the war toward matters of race, nationality, and immigration was an ambiguous one, a curious mixture of optimism and pessimism. A large number still believed in the assimilative powers of the American environment, but to many others the idea of the melting pot had already been exposed as a myth. Anti-immigrant sentiment was common to the progressives, but they disagreed among themselves as to whether the answer was restriction, as E. A. Ross suggested, or assimilation, as Jane Addams advised. Theodore Roosevelt's chauvinism and jingoism symbolized one side of the American mood; his fear of the "Yellow Peril" and of "race suicide" symbolized the other. Throughout this period the immigrant was in a difficult position. Politically, most immigrants were deeply conservative; very few ever became socialists or radicals. Many radical leaders, most notably Eugene Debs and Norman Thomas, were in fact native-born, middle-class Americans. Nevertheless, most of the truly radical movements in the United States at the end of the nineteenth and the beginning of the twentieth century were populated largely by recent immigrants. All of the various socialist parties, including that of Debs, had a very large ingredient of immigrants actually organized in foreign-language units. Accordingly, since the time of the Haymarket affair in 1886, no general stereotype of the immigrant prevailed more than that of a lawless creature, prone to radicalism, anarchy, and violence. Similarly, many looked disdainfully upon immigrants for not assimilating fast enough, but the greatest hostility before the outbreak of the war tended to be directed at those immigrant groups which were most rapidly climbing up the social scale.[32] Some of those who in word criticized

32. John Higham, "Another Look at Nativism," *Catholic Historical Review*, 44(1958):151–58.

immigrants for not assimilating in deed often prevented them from doing so: they urged Americanization, but created the social register and the patriotic society; they urged assimilation, but moved elsewhere when immigrants acquired the means to move into their neighborhoods and churches. "The native American is too proud to mix socially with them,"[33] Grant wrote haughtily. Anti-immigrant sentiment at this time tended to be primarily verbal—with the exception of a few zealots like the hard-line eugenicists and the members of the Immigration Restriction League, few people thought in terms of legislation—but it indicated the existence of a general mood which potentially could develop into a more intense hostility. The number of individuals at the start of World War I who desired to have immigration restricted was far from small, but such persons would not yet have dared to predict that they would achieve resounding victory within a decade.

After the war, many individuals for the first time began to regard the incoming tide with great horror. Foremost among the reasons for this were the economic considerations mentioned earlier, but there were other factors as well. As shipping which had been detained for military purposes became available to transport civilians, immigration, which had virtually ceased during the war, began to rise rapidly.[34] Immigrants and colored races had performed relatively poorly on the first Stanford-Binet intelligence test in 1916, a fact racists promptly seized as "proof" of the inherently inferior mental capacities of these groups. Anthropology, with the significant exception of the work done by Franz Boas, was providing little evidence to counter racist propaganda; anthropologists at this time had not reached a consensus as to what constitutes a racial trait, and they had not

33. Madison Grant, *The Passing of the Great Race* (New York: Charles Scribner's Sons, 1916), p. 80.
34. Immigration statistics for the decade between 1912 and 1921, from the *Annual Reports of the Commissioner General of Immigration:*

Year	Alien Immigrants to the United States
1912	838,172
1913	1,197,892
1914	1,218,480
1915	326,700
1916	298,826
1917	295,403
1918	110,618
1919	141,132
1920	430,001
1921	805,228

yet begun to appreciate the relevance of genetic findings for their own work.[35] The country was caught up in post-war waves of nationalism and isolationism and entertained a marked distrust of anything foreign. Public indignation toward "hyphenated" Americans, aroused by Theodore Roosevelt during the war, was still acute; many suspected that immigrants were loyal to their old homelands rather than to America (despite the fact that during the war 450,000 foreign-born men ineligible for the draft had volunteered for service). The country was swept by the "Red Scare" of the post-war period, and it was commonly feared that immigrants were falling prey to communism, anarchism, and radicalism. Many Americans were deeply troubled that millions of Communists would enter the United States as agents of the recently triumphant Bolshevik Revolution in Russia. Waves of anti-Semitism and anti-Catholicism accentuated the hostility toward the newcomers; so also did a series of labor strikes in the early 1920's in which immigrants played prominent roles. The notion of the frontier "escape valve" was now only a memory.[36] The result of all these factors was the development of an anti-immigration sentiment which found legislative expression in the 1921 Immigration Act.

The 1921 act was only a temporary law; industry and the steamship companies lobbied effectively enough to prevent permanent legislation from being enacted. Soon after this bill was passed, however, genetic and racial arguments replaced economic considerations as the most conspicuous feature of the immigration debates. Proponents of restriction employed genetic theories to justify the claim that southern and eastern European immigrants were "biologically inferior" peoples. This argument was effective since it could appeal to the intense animosities toward foreigners and immigrants which had been produced by the war. It enabled restrictionists to guise their hostilities toward minorities with an apparent scientific blessing. Its foremost advocates were eugenicists, who forcefully and repeatedly presented it to both Congress and the general public.

35. Some geneticists at this time expressed disappointment at anthropologists' lack of familiarity with their work. As Davenport remarked: "I think the future will find it almost inexplicable that now, 15 years after the proper way of looking at heredity and 'species' or 'races' has been made clear there are not half a dozen anthropologists who make use of the new point of view." (Charles B. Davenport to Aleš Hrdlička, May 5, 1915, CBD.)

36. Some have argued that the frontier "escape valve" existed more in the mind than in reality as part of the nineteenth century social scene. Ray Allen Billington, in his work Westward Expansion (New York: Macmillan, 1949), challenges the "escape valve" thesis—at least as soon as the frontier ceased to be around the bend of the river or just over the horizon. Billington calculated (p. 10) that a modest homestead in the 1850's would require at least $1,500 to establish. Such expenses effectively barred the poor from participating in any "escape."

In abbreviated form, the eugenicists' biological argument against the "new" immigration involved two parts. First, they labeled the "new" immigrant as genetically inferior to the "Nordic" or "American" or "Anglo-Saxon" type. This was generally done by invoking the Social Darwinistic assumption that a person's economic and social status is indicative of his hereditary worth. To eugenicists the high incidence of disease, illiteracy, poverty, and crime in immigrant neighborhoods constituted sufficient testimony to the newcomers' innate inferiority.[37] In addition, eugenicists advanced two propositions about genetics. They maintained that heredity is far more important than environment—an assumption which justified their claim that immigrants' "undesirable" features could in no way be corrected or improved. Further, they cited the theory of "disharmonious crossings," the view that the offspring of a cross between two different strains will always be inferior to both parental strains. With this theory, the eugenicists asserted that "American" blood was incompatible with foreign blood, that any mixing between the two would destroy the quality of the country's native stock. Using these arguments, eugenicists campaigned energetically for *selective* immigration restriction to guard the nation's racial homogeneity.

This position was expounded most forcefully by Laughlin. In April, 1920, he had been appointed the "expert eugenics agent" of the House Committee on Immigration and Naturalization, and during the debates over immigration restriction, he appeared before the committee on several occasions, always presenting the view that the biologically inferior new immigration was threatening to wipe out the native American stock. The widely quoted conclusion from his most important testimony, "Analysis of America's Modern Melting Pot" (1922) was: "Making all logical allowances for environmental conditions, which may be unfavorable to the immigrant, the recent immigrants, as a whole, present a higher percentage of inborn socially inadequate qualities than do the older stocks."[38] This view was restated in his important 1924 testimony before the House Committee, "Europe as an Emigrant-Exporting Continent."

Laughlin's conclusions were based upon a biased interpretation of statistical evidence and the eugenic assumptions about biology.[39] Even judged

37. Carroll Ann Smith discusses these arguments in detail in "Anglo-Saxon Science: The Scientific Rationale for Immigration Restriction" (Columbia University, unpublished Master's Thesis, 1958).

38. Harry H. Laughlin, "Analysis of America's Modern Melting Pot," *Hearings before the House Committee on Immigration and Naturalization*, 67th Congress, 3rd Session (Washington: Government Printing Office, 1922), p. 755.

39. Oscar Handlin exposes the inaccuracy and illogic of the Laughlin report in *Race and Nationality in American Life* (Boston: Little, Brown and Co., 1957), chapter 5.

by the biological knowledge of the day, his interpretations were faulty, his claims unfounded. The role of environment had been firmly recognized; the theory that all crossings between strains are "disharmonious" had been discredited; and no reputable geneticist would have dared to judge a person's "genetic worth" by his social standing alone. In the early 1920's, however, virtually no geneticist or biologist of note publicly contradicted Laughlin's work. Thus, what gave his reports so much influence was that the public *thought* they were unbiased and scientifically accurate. Many accepted his professions of objectivity and disinterest, such as this one:

> I made this biological investigation ["Europe as an Emigrant-Exporting Continent"] and put the facts on record here for the benefit of the committee, which must draw its own conclusions. I am not here as an advocate for or against any race. Indeed, my position with the Carnegie Institution of Washington would prevent me from standing as an advocate or special pleader.
> I must state also that as a member of the Carnegie Institution of Washington, if I were biased in favor of the immediate financial interests that created the institution, I should perhaps advocate open immigration in order to get cheaper labor, which might increase the immediate profits of Carnegie investments. But I am not doing that. I am here simply as a scientific investigator to present the facts to the gentlemen of the committee, with the hope that the facts and their analysis might be of use.[40]

Declaring that immigration was a biological rather than an economic problem, he continually stressed his "non-partisan" interest in the issue:

> For the Nation to permit any vested interest, domestic or foreign, to dominate its immigration policy for a long time would bring certain disaster. The economic policy, as I have often said in this report, is giving way in the United States to the biological, which weighs primarily the future basic or family stock welfare of the whole Nation. If, because of these reports, those who favor a restriction of numbers and a rigid selection of immigrants have found more ammunition than those who favor open immigration, that is a sequence for which the investigator is not responsible.[41]

Laughlin's reports epitomized the eugenic argument for immigration restriction and had a far-reaching impact upon Congressmen during the immigration debates. One opponent of restriction, Bruno Lasker, editor of *The Survey*, bemoaned: "We feel that Dr. Laughlin's arguments for further

40. Harry H. Laughlin, "Europe as an Emigrant-Exporting Continent," *Hearings before the House Committee on Immigration and Naturalization*, 68th Congress, 1st Session (Washington: Government Printing Office, 1924), p. 1318.
41. *Ibid.*, p. 1306.

restriction are difficult to combat if they are true, and that his facts will in the future be thrown at us every time we plead for liberal treatment of the immigration question."[42] That indeed happened. Throughout the discussion of the immigration issue, Laughlin was widely quoted and praised by members of both branches of Congress. Representative Albert Johnson of Washington, Chairman of the House Committee on Immigration and Naturalization, spoke for many members of Congress when he called the "Melting Pot" "one of the most valuable documents ever put out by a committee of Congress."[43]

Although the "Melting Pot" appeared in 1922, the majority opinion was not yet in favor of a "biological" immigration bill. In 1923 Johnson presented to Congress a measure which called for immigration to be restricted to two per cent of the 1890 census, but the bill failed. While Johnson continued to consolidate support in Congress, many eugenicists and their sympathizers carried the "biological" arguments to the popular press. Grant's book went into a new edition in 1921; Lothrop Stoddard published *The Rising Tide of Color* in 1920 and *The Racial Realities in Europe* in 1924; Kenneth Roberts and Gino Speranza wrote a series of influential articles in popular magazines in 1923 and 1924; Prescott Hall and Robert DeC. Ward lectured and wrote on the topic repeatedly. These efforts helped muster further public sentiment in favor of selective restriction. The clamor prompted one supporter to write Johnson: "Since much stress has been laid upon the less desirable features of the races coming from the southern and eastern parts of Europe and the parts of the nearer west, I believe that the change to the 1890 census is absolutely necessary."[44] Another feared: "We are rapidly losing ground to the emotional foreigner who is biologically unlike us and therefore cannot understand that honesty, loyalty, and moral life are principles inherent in good minds."[45] Still another one insisted: "Inferior stock shall not populate our country and reproduce imbecility, feeble-mindedness and criminality with its subdiary [sic], prostitution. Now it has been proven that prostitution and criminality is a matter of either heredity or environment. But heredity is the main cause."[46]

By late fall of 1923, the public demand for a "biological" restriction law had become overwhelming. Grant told Johnson: "I believe you have the country behind you and a most popular cause. It is growing in strength

42. Bruno Lasker to Herbert S. Jennings, November 24, 1923, *HSJ*.
43. *Congressional Record* (April 5, 1924), p. 5648.
44. H. M. Allen to Albert Johnson, January 21, 1924, *Correspondence*.
45. Mrs. Mary Brown to Albert Johnson, February 9, 1924, *Correspondence*.
46. William Lee Corey to Albert Johnson, July 24, 1924, *Correspondence*.

every day and it is only a question of time when even greater restrictive measures will be put through."[47] Supporters of such a law had received the unofficial endorsement of both President Calvin Coolidge and Secretary of Labor James J. Davis. Writing in *Good Housekeeping*, Coolidge had stated: "There are racial considerations too grave to be brushed aside for any sentimental reasons. Biological laws tell us that certain divergent people will not mix or blend. The Nordics propagate themselves successfully. With other races, the outcome shows deterioration on both sides. Quality of mind and body suggests that observance of ethnic law is as great a necessity to a nation as immigration law."[48] Davis, an admirer of Laughlin's work,[49] believed that "America has always prided itself upon having for its basic stock the so-called 'Nordic races'."[50] He had urged that "we should bar from our shores all races which are not naturalizable under the law of the land and all individuals of all races who are physically, mentally, morally and spiritually undesirable, and who constitute a menace to our civilization."[51] As the 68th Congress prepared to open in December, Johnson began mapping strategy for his immigration bill.

Soon after Congress convened, attention turned to the public hearings on the immigration issue held by the House and Senate Committees on Immigration. These hearings served as an arena for individuals and organizations representing both sides of the immigration question. Spokesmen for labor, patriotic societies, fraternal groups, and eugenic organizations testified on behalf of the bill; representatives of industry, steamship companies, agriculture, and immigrant aid societies argued against it.[52] The same vested interests that had battled to a deadlock in 1921 were still in contention.

During the Senate hearings, biological arguments were only occasionally heard, and the committee devoted much of its attention to the fine points

47. Madison Grant to Albert Johnson, December 22, 1923, *Correspondence*.
48. Calvin Coolidge, "Whose Country Is This?" *Good Housekeeping,* 72 (February, 1921):14.
49. James J. Davis, "Our Labor Shortage and Immigration," *Industrial Management,* 65(1923):321.
50. *Ibid.*, p. 322.
51. *Ibid.*, p. 323.
52. For several reasons industry opposed the 1924 bill less vigorously than the 1921 measure. During the intervening three years the popular fear of the racial effects of immigration had heightened, business had continued to prosper even without its former supply of cheap labor, and a major new source of labor had been provided by large-scale Negro migration to the industrial North.
Not all members of minority groups opposed the 1924 bill. In particular, those who considered themselves to be "Americanized" because of their pre-Civil War American ancestry sometimes sided with the restrictionists. In what seems to have

of administering the proposed legislation. There were two reasons for its concern with details. First, the Senate hearings were held after the House hearings and very shortly before the immigration issue was scheduled to be brought to the Congressional floor. Having read the House testimony, the members of the Senate committee had already digested the racial aspects of that debate.[53] Moreover, compared with their counterparts in the House, some members of the Senate committee were unsympathetic toward the biological argument. In particular, the tolerance toward minorities shown by Senator LeBaron B. Colt of Rhode Island, chairman of the committee, who felt that "when you discriminate markedly against any group you are raising racial antagonism, which is entirely un-American,"[54] placed him in marked contrast to Johnson. On several occasions Johnson himself expressed the fear that the Senate committee would delay his proposed bill.[55] His suspicions were justified, for the Senate committee finally voted *against* the selective restriction clause and offered the Senate a measure which would limit restriction to two per cent of the *1910* census.

During the House hearings, however, genetic arguments for selective restriction were prominent. Citizens and Congressmen both appeared before the committee to testify that "biology" demanded the immediate enactment of such a measure. One of the most important speeches before the committee was that of Thomas W. Phillips, a representative from Pennsylvania, a man of the view that "whether our civilization can be advanced or even maintained will depend upon the quality of its human supporters,

---

been an effort to reaffirm their own sense of belonging, they labeled the newcomers as outsiders—even those of the same ethnic origin. As discussion of the Johnson bill was proceeding, one such individual, a self-proclaimed "secretary of six organizations, including the local Republican organization of this district," wrote to Johnson on stationary of the "Actors and Authors League" to "voice my most emphatic approval of the Immigration bill now pending in Congress, bearing your name." He stated: "As an American Hebrew I do not regard the bill at all prejudicial to members of my faith, the repeated cries of several of the so-called Jewish leaders notwithstanding." Of the Jewish district in which he lived, he said: "In my neighborhood I seldom hear the English language spoken. The merchants of this vicinity have nearly all their merchandise labeled in Yiddish. I do not know whether I am getting a can of salmon or a box of Babbits cleaner." He regretted the lack of support given selective restriction by his neighbors, complaining: "They do not vote like Americans." (Milton B. Benjamin to Albert Johnson, February 21, 1924, *Correspondence.*)

53. "Selective Immigration Legislation," *Hearings Before the Senate Committee on Immigration*, 68th Congress, 1st Session (Washington: Government Printing Office, 1924), p. 73.

54. *Ibid.*, p. 75.

55. See Albert Johnson to John D. Currie, March 10, 1924; and Mrs. J. S. McKee to Editor of *The Oregonian*, February 24, 1924; both *Correspondence.*

and quality depends largely upon inheritance."[56] Phillips told the committee members:

> We know better than to import vicious or refractory domestic animals but, on the contrary, through intelligent and careful selection from abroad, bend every effort to improve our home stock of domestic animals. . . .
> We must set up artificial means through legal machinery to hand pick our immigrants if we are going to prevent rapid deterioration of our citizenship. The immigration law should be sufficiently elastic to permit those charged with its enforcement to apply any present or future knowledge of biology, in so far as such knowledge throws light on the results that follow the mating of individuals of different races or individuals of widely separated branches of the same race.[57]

Proponents of this view found a receptive audience in the members of the House Committee. Though critics of Laughlin and his "racial biology" also appeared at the hearings, their objections were treated lightly; the committee members preferred to quote Laughlin rather than to challenge him. As committeeman John C. Box of Texas stated: "One cardinal principle which has controlled the committee in providing this additional method of selection [1890 as census year] is the consideration of racial homogeneity."[58] After concluding the hearings, the committee voted by a 15 to 2 margin to send the Johnson bill to the floor. Only Adolph J. Sabath and Samuel Dickstein, both Jews, voted against the bill in committee. Dickstein complained soon afterwards, "If you had been a member of that committee you could not help but understand that they did not want anybody else in this country except the Nordics."[59]

Once discussion of the Johnson bill opened on the floors of Congress, the impact of these genetic arguments was readily discernible. In both the House and the Senate, biological and racial argument dominated the debate. Representative Robert Allen of West Virginia stated: "The primary reason for the restriction of the alien stream, however, is the necessity for purifying and keeping pure the blood of America."[60] Representative Grant Hudson of Michigan added: "We are slowly awakening to the conscious-

56. "Restriction of Immigration," *Hearings before the House Committee on Immigration and Naturalization*, 68th Congress, 1st Session (Washington: Government Printing Office, 1924), p. 768.

57. *Ibid.*, pp. 767-68.

58. *Congressional Record* (April 8, 1924), p. 5876.

59. *Ibid.* (April 5, 1924), p. 5687.

60. *Ibid.* (April 5, 1924), p. 5693.

ness that education and environment do not fundamentally alter racial values."[61] Senator Henry Ashurst of Arizona, temporarily digressing to discuss Oriental immigrants, declared: "Against the Japanese and their civilization I have no evil word, but we are a different race. They will vitiate our population, and once it is vitiated it is beyond repair."[62] Representative J. Will Taylor of Tennessee quoted a letter "which impressed me with its logic and philosophy": "America is slipping and sinking as Rome did, and from identical causes. Rome had faith in the melting pot, as we have. It scorned the iron certainties of heredity, as we do. It lost its instinct for race preservation, as we have lost ours."[63]

Debate over the bill was furious; opponents voiced strident criticisms; but in the end, both in the House and the Senate, it passed by large majorities. Virtually the sole opposition came from the northeastern states, where immigrant groups in the cities were well-organized politically. Party affiliation was apparently not a factor, for in the House the bill was opposed by 35 Republicans and 36 Democrats. The act was a popular measure, and it was widely hailed for its "biological wisdom." Eugenicists were exultant. "It is a matter for congratulation that the United States now bases its immigration policy upon the eugenic quality of the racial stock, and attempts to exclude undesirable racial stock,"[64] Clarence G. Campbell stated in his presidential address to the Eugenics Research Association. "It [the Johnson Act] expressed the conviction of the American people that immigration is a long-time investment in family stocks rather than a short-time investment in productive labor,"[65] Ward wrote. "This victory should make you senator!"[66] Grant exclaimed to Johnson.

Genetic theory thus played a crucial role in the passage of the 1924 Immigration Restriction Act. As discussed in Chapter 2, nevertheless, the commitment of many of the spokesmen for eugenic immigration policy was not to scientific truth, as they said so often in public, but to the justification of their violent prejudices against the newcomers. To such men the biological argument appealed greatly, for it provided their views a cloak of scientific authority. So useful to them was eugenic theory that at one time the officers of the Immigration Restriction League had even

61. *Ibid.* (April 5, 1924), p. 5641.
62. *Ibid.* (April 8, 1924), p. 5825.
63. *Ibid.* (April 8, 1924), p. 5872.
64. Clarence G. Campbell, "Presidential Address of the Eugenics Research Association: Positive Eugenics," *Eugenical News*, 14(1929):93.
65. Robert DeC. Ward, "The New Immigration Law and its Operation," *Scientific Monthly*, 21(1925):53.
66. Madison Grant to Albert Johnson, April 17, 1924, *Correspondence.*

considered changing the organization's name to the "Eugenic Immigration League."[67]

In Congress, eugenicists had their greatest influence on Johnson himself. A former small-town newspaper publisher, he had gotten his start in politics by leading an anti-radicalism crusade directed against the radical labor group, the International Workers of the World. Elected to Congress in 1912 and chairman of the House Committee on Immigration and Naturalization since 1919, he enthusiastically endorsed eugenic arguments for immigration restriction, and he continually enlisted the aid of eugenicists when planning legislation on the matter. "I sincerely hope that the eugenics feature as applicable to immigration may be carefully developed and continually pressed,"[68] he told Irving Fisher. In the fall of 1923 he discussed the immigration issue with the Eugenics Committee of the United States of America, and that winter he collaborated with the Eugenics Committee in order to co-ordinate their publicity efforts on behalf of his bill.[69] In 1924 he was in correspondence with the eugenicist Henry Pratt Fairchild over how "to find a basis for regulating immigration which would secure the result which every sensible American wants, and yet be free from the charge of unfair and arbitrary discrimination to which, however unjustifiably, the use of the 1890 census is susceptible."[70] He mixed socially with eugenicists and became the close personal friend of Grant, Laughlin, Ward, Fairchild, and others.[71] In 1923 he even became a member of the Immigration Subcommittee of the Eugenics Committee of the United States of America. That same year, in honor of his many "services" to the cause of eugenics, he was elected honorary president of the Eugenics Research Association. Laughlin called him "the great American watchdog whose job it is to protect the blood of the American people from contamination and degeneracy."[72]

An emphatic man, dogmatic, chauvinistic, extremely prejudiced against aliens, Johnson became committed to eugenic arguments and would not

67. Higham, *Strangers in the Land*, p. 152.

68. Albert Johnson to Irving Fisher, May 1, 1923, *Correspondence*.

69. See Johnson's correspondence with Irving Fisher and Robert DeC. Ward, *Correspondence*.

70. Henry Pratt Fairchild to Albert Johnson, April 15, 1924; see also Johnson to Fairchild, April 17, 1924; both *Correspondence*.

71. Johnson's correspondence includes mention of several occasions in which he met eugenicists socially. He seemed particularly attracted to Grant and would visit him whenever possible. Though Grant held no elected or appointed public office, Johnson usually would address letters to him as "The Honorable Madison Grant." See *Correspondence*.

72. "Eugenics in America," text of a lecture presented by Laughlin to the Eugenics Education Society in London, Tuesday, January 29, 1924, *Correspondence*.

tolerate any criticism of them. *Prior* to the immigration hearings held by his committee, he felt that the biological questions of immigration "have been settled in the minds of members of the House and Senate."[73] A few months later he wrote: "My experience is that all earnest minded citizens who have studied the subject from the viewpoint of the United States, present and future, once they become attached to 1890 as a quota base for the regulation of immigration, are unable to detach themselves therefrom. *The thing admits of no argument*"[74] [italics mine]. During his committee's hearings he ignored those who denounced the Laughlin Report. When Laughlin complained of being criticized, the chairman replied: "Don't worry about criticism, Doctor Laughlin, you have developed a valuable research and demonstrated a most startling state of affairs. We shall pursue these biological studies further."[75]

Johnson's emotional commitment to eugenic theories was shared by other members of the House Immigration Committee. When one opponent of restriction criticized "The Melting Pot," John C. Box lost control of his temper; he heatedly accused the man of attacking the report for economic gain, without pausing to weigh the merits of what the man had said.[76] Arthur M. Free of California, who had been a student of E. A. Ross at Stanford, desired to learn his former professor's opinions of immigration. "I am indeed pleased to get your views on the matter and assure you I will be pleased to hear from you at any future time on this and any other subject,"[77] the congressman wrote. Ross, it will be remembered, was still enchanted with the idea of Nordic supremacy. Like some eugenicists, these congressmen seemed motivated by prejudice. A quotation from John N. Vaile of Colorado is illustrative:

Let me emphasize here that the "restrictionists" of Congress do not claim that the "Nordic" race, or even the Anglo-Saxon race, is the best race in the world. Let us concede, in all fairness, that the Czech is a more sturdy laborer, with very low percentage of crime and insanity, that the Jew is the best business man in the world, and that the Italian has a spiritual grasp and an artistic sense which have greatly enriched the world and which have, indeed, enriched us, a spiritual exaltation and an artistic creative sense which the Nordic rarely attains. Nordics need not be vain about their own qualifications. It well behooves them to be humble. What we do claim is that the northern European, and particularly Anglo-Saxons,

73. Albert Johnson to Captain John B. Trevor, December 8, 1923, *Correspondence.*
74. Albert Johnson to Frederick F. Schrader, March 12, 1924, *Correspondence.*
75. Laughlin, "Europe as an Emigrant-Exporting Continent," p. 1311.
76. "Restriction of Immigration," pp. 272-74.
77. A. M. Free to E. A. Ross, February 1, 1927, *EAR.*

made this country. Oh, yes; the others helped. But that is the full statement of the case. They came to this country because it was already made
as an Anglo-Saxon commonwealth. They added to it, they often enriched
it, but they did not make it, and they have not yet greatly changed it. We
are determined that they shall not. It is a good country. It suits us. And
what we assert is that we are not going to surrender it to somebody else or
allow other people, no matter what their merits, to make it something
different. If there is any changing to be done, we will do it ourselves.[78]

Deeply prejudiced against immigrants, the House Committee members
summoned persons of similar views to the hearings. Ward, Grant,
Stoddard, Speranza, and Roberts—but no biologists of standing—were requested to appear. The only geneticist who finally did testify before the
committee, H. S. Jennings, received a belated, begrudging invitation. Originally Johnson had not intended to include him, but later he did so in order
to mitigate the complaints of Representative Emanuel Celler of New York
that the committee's selection of witnesses was biased. Jennings was
crowded into the afternoon session of Friday, January 4, 1924, with five
other speakers. Offered only a few minutes of the committee's time, he
was told not to present his case then but to submit a written report. A
Johnson memorandum to Jennings the following Wednesday stated that
the chairman "regrets exceedingly"[79] that Jennings was brought to the
hearings on a day already crowded with witnesses. Such was the treatment
given the one man whom even Laughlin later was to deem worthy of a
reply!
  Prejudice in Congress was not limited to members of the House Immigration Committee. Representative Walter Lineberger of California complained to Johnson that a certain section of Los Angeles "has been over-
run as with a swarm of ants, by a multitude of Jewish junk men, peddlers,
and what not, in sickening contrast to the Anglo-Saxon inhabitants of the
earlier time."[80] As a freshman representative during the 68th Congress,
Celler, the current chairman of the House Judiciary Committee and long a
foe of the national origins principle, was shocked by the prevalence of
such views. Many representatives, from rural areas particularly, would
casually call foreigners by the most derogatory epithets. The dominant
attitude in Congress was that one "race" was better than another; the great
majority of legislators accepted the eugenicists' claim that this was the
dictate of science. Such ideas revolted Celler and put him avidly on the
side of the anti-restrictionists. He felt like a lone voice in the wilderness,

  78. *Congressional Record* (April 8, 1924), p. 5922.
  79. Albert Johnson to H. S. Jennings, January 9, 1924, *Correspondence.*
  80. Walter F. Lineberger to Albert Johnson, December 18, 1923, *Correspondence.*

since Johnson's control of the immigration matter in Congress was complete.[81]

Laughlin himself was the individual most biased in his views and least tolerant of criticism. Rather than answering objections to his work, he ridiculed his critics and bragged of his "scientific authority." "The only criticism which I must take most seriously is that of Prof. H. S. Jennings, of Johns Hopkins,"[82] he said; and by a remarkable twist of logic he found Jennings in agreement with him. Jennings in fact had appeared before the House Committee to impugn Laughlin's conclusions! The other critics, as far as he was concerned, were merely bitter losers. "If the facts had turned the conclusions in another direction," he declared, "I doubt not that the present critics would have been silent."[83] "When the criticism is made by a person who has never conducted studies of this sort and who tries to predict what he would find if researches were made in a certain way, and who calls the present studies biased, and who is trying, apparently, to count out the value of the study because its conclusions are displeasing to him, the scientific investigator must, despite his joy in a good fight, ignore petty heckling."[84]

The bias of the House Committee and some of its allies did not escape the notice of critics in Congress. Sabath claimed: "They believe these people are inferior. They have been fed by misinformation; they have been fed by new dope, as I may term it, by unreliable statisticians, and by Professor Laughlin's eugenic and anthropological false tests, until they themselves believe that there is some foundation for the unjustifiable conclusions contained in the so-called Laughlin report."[85] Celler complained:

We have heard a great deal in the discussions of the subject of races, race types, ethnic strains, heredity, germ plasms, and so forth. What efforts were made by the committee to know something of the important phases of the subject? Instead of calling Lothrop Stoddard and Madison Grant, why did they not call Dr. Ales Hrdlicka, curator of physical anthropology, National Museum at Washington, D. C.? Doctor Hrdlicka is well known to the chairman of the committee. . . . No; the committee only wanted those who believed in 'Nordic' superiority; men who deal in buncombe, like Grant and Stoddard.[86]

Representative Patrick O'Sullivan of Connecticut asserted: "In the background of this doctrine of the inferiority of the southern European a

81. Conversation with Emanuel Celler, July 14, 1971.
82. Laughlin, "Europe as an Emigrant-Exporting Continent," p. 1316.
83. *Ibid.*, p. 1311.
84. *Ibid.*, p. 1317.
85. *Congressional Record* (April 5, 1924), p. 5662.
86. *Ibid.* (April 8, 1924), p. 5915.

rather extraordinary fiction is built relating to a race known as the Nordic, which appears to have been quite overlooked by anthropologists until recently."[87] In the face of such severe criticism, how was the Johnson bill able to achieve such an overwhelming victory?

For one thing, congressmen responded to the restrictionist sentiment of the times. The desire to limit immigration was already present; biology merely justified it further and directed its legislative form. It is difficult today to appreciate the profound anxiety of the early 1920's and the degree to which immigrants served as a convenient explanation for America's ills. Johnson's correspondence from private citizens provides one indication of this. Some wrote to him accusing immigrants of not Americanizing fast enough ("Millions are yet unassimilated, un-Americanized and intend, with untiring efforts, only to gain the coveted amount sufficient to take them back to the land of their birth"[88]); whereas others criticized the newcomers for assimilating too rapidly ("New York is being captured ten fold more effectively by foreigners even less desirable than the Germans would have been as a conquering enemy"[89]). Immigrants were objects of vicious calumny, particularly from native-born citizens of Anglo-Saxon stock writing from urban centers of high immigrant concentration. If she were not speaking seriously, one woman's fear of foreigners would seem even more ludicrous than it already does: "Our beloved America is being taken away from us by Asiatics, Japs, and other horrible European people: why the Italians and Jews are about eating us up. If there are any Japs around please destroy this letter as I am deadly afraid of them."[90] Addressing a meeting of eugenicists in 1928, Johnson described the feeling which was prevalent among many: "Had we not imposed a drastic inhibition upon a world migration to our shores, what we know as the American people and its institutions would have been submerged in chaos."[91]

It was in this social context, then, that principles of biology proved to be an effective weapon against immigration. Most supporters of restriction, in and out of Congress, were not so hysterically prejudiced as many leaders of the campaign; but, immersed in the anxieties of the age, they accepted the biological arguments uncritically. Even the unprejudiced supporters did not realize that the "biology" they were using was a misrepresentation

87. *Ibid.* (April 8, 1924), p. 5899.
88. W. D. Thompson (and 9 others) to Albert Johnson, March 11, 1924, *Correspondence.*
89. J. A. Webb to Albert Johnson, January 24, 1925, *Correspondence.*
90. Mrs. Eva E. Martin to Albert Johnson, April, 1924, *Correspondence.*
91. Albert Johnson, "The Menace of the Melting Pot Myth," in *Proceedings of the Third Race Betterment Conference* (Battle Creek, Michigan: The Race Betterment Foundation, 1928), p. 200.

of the existing state of knowledge. Only after Hitler achieved power, when the full implications of "eugenic schemes" became generally recognized, did many supporters of a biological immigration law become vocal opponents of hereditary deterministic explanations of human nature.

In addition, while the Johnson bill was being debated, assertions by eugenicists were not being countered by persons of authority within genetics. Of the thousands of letters received by Johnson while his measure was pending, not one was from a geneticist or biologist, though several dozen were from important eugenicists. Jennings, the one geneticist who testified during the 68th Congress, entered the fray only at the last minute, too late to sway many minds. Raymond Pearl was correct when he told Jennings:

> Without having gone at all deeply into the matter, I have had a strong feeling that the reactionary group led by Madison Grant and with Laughlin as its chief spade worker were likely, in their zeal for the Nordic, to do a great deal of real harm. So far as I can learn, there is no other group which makes the least pretension to being scientific which is interesting itself in any practical way in this pending immigration legislation. From what I hear, I judge that the opinions of Congressmen generally regarding this group is that it is the only one which has any scientific knowledge about immigration.[92]

Thus, eugenicists' authority was effective and uncontested during the course of the immigration debates. Genetic theory gave their view a scientific sanction which opponents could not combat; it made the selective restriction against the new immigration seem like a biological imperative. Operating on the deep anxieties and prejudices toward foreigners and immigrants which had been fostered by World War I, it enabled restrictionists to mask their hatreds under a veneer of scientific objectivity. With "genetic truth" as a motto, their forces swept to victory. Though afterwards many geneticists were to look upon these events with deep regret, nevertheless they were soon to witness in Germany a still more immense perversion of their science.

3. Eugenics in Nazi Germany

The German eugenics movement, like similar movements elsewhere, began at the turn of the century. The most important eugenics society, the Deutsche Gesellschaft für Rassenhygiene, was established in 1902; the major eugenics journal, the *Archiv für Rassen- und Gesellschaftsbiologie* was founded in 1903. From the start eugenics in Germany was character-

---

92. Raymond Pearl to Herbert S. Jennings, November 24, 1923, *HSJ.*

ized by the same mixture of objective and biased research as in other countries. The movement boasted as members eminent scientists—Wilhelm Weinberg discussed the eugenic implications of his findings in a number of his papers and served for many years as chairman of the Stuttgart chapter of the Deutsche Gesellschaft für Rassenhygiene[93]—but it also attracted many prejudiced persons. Some German eugenicists seemed to be oriented toward both the scientific and pseudoscientific. Eugen Fischer, who became a leading exponent of Nazi Aryanism and a prominent official of the Third Reich, was also an internationally respected geneticist and anthropologist.[94]

The English edition (1931) of *Human Heredity* by Erwin Baur, Eugen Fischer, and Fritz Lenz dramatically illustrated the confusion of purpose within German eugenics and human genetics. All three authors were prominent biologists, though Lenz and Fischer were also major contributors to the pseudoscientific literature on race and eugenics. Lenz was an outright anti-Semite, while Fischer eventually became a Nazi official. The book was read widely, both in Germany and throughout the world, and it was commonly said that an earlier edition had greatly influenced Hitler while he was in prison writing *Mein Kampf*.[95] Though more than one American biologist considered it to be "the best existing book on human inheritance,"[96] the authors themselves insisted that its primary purpose was merely to provide the theoretical foundation for a later volume on eugenics.[97]

The volume began innocently enough. Baur's opening presentation of basic genetic principles was written soundly and objectively. Even so critical a reviewer as H. J. Muller praised this discussion ("We would commend this section of the book highly, along with everything else that has issued from Baur's pen,"[98] he wrote) as he also praised Lenz's chapter on meth-

93. Curt Stern, "Wilhelm Weinberg," *Genetics*, 47(1962):4.

94. Not all areas of genetics or human genetics are of equal social import; often it is easier to approach objectively problems of minor social significance. In 1912 Fischer performed an excellent study of race crossing among Hottentots, but surely the study of Hottentots was a topic far less socially explosive than the investigation of the mental traits of the major European "races"!

95. H. J. Muller, "Human Heredity," *Birth Control Review*, 17(1933):21; Paul Popenoe, "The German Sterilization Law," *Journal of Heredity*, 25(1934):257. Most experts consider Adolf Hitler's "imprisonment" for a few months somewhat of a farce. He was allowed visitors without limit. It would appear that he dictated *Mein Kampf* to Rudolf Hess during this "confinement" at Landsberg prison. Nine months' confinement for conviction of high treason was indeed a light sentence!

96. "Menschliche Erblichkeitslehre und Rassenhygiene," *The Quarterly Review of Biology*, 3(1928):136; Muller, "Human Heredity," p. 19.

97. Erwin Baur, Eugen Fischer, and Fritz Lenz, *Human Heredity*, 3rd ed., trans. by Eden and Cedar Paul (London: George Allen & Unwin, 1931), p. 20.

98. Muller, "Human Heredity," p. 19.

odology. However, the sections by Fischer and Lenz on physical and mental differences among "races" deviated sharply from the high standard established by Baur. Forgetting that earlier they had acknowledged the importance of environment as well as heredity in the development of human characteristics, they proceeded to interpret almost all superficial differences among ethnic groups as being genetic in origin, thereby giving "scientific" credence to the popular stereotypes of "inferior" non-"Nordic" races. ("What a curious coincidence, that Lenz and Fischer should both be Nordics!"[99] Muller exclaimed.) In ominously foreboding words Lenz spoke of "the Jewish problem," claiming: "It is true that whereas the Teutons could get along fairly well without the Jews, the Jews could not get along without the Teutons."[100] The most portentous statement of the book came in the authors' preface:

> Comparatively little change has been requisite in Baur's section, dealing with the general theory of heredity, for in this department the elements of our science have been fairly well stabilised. But even in the more specialized field of human heredity, a like stabilisation is already in progress, so that we may hope that future editions of this book will not need so radical a revision.[101]

Perhaps this prediction of a "stabilization" of knowledge was a scientific misjudgment on their part. On the other hand, perhaps it marked the point where human genetics in Germany became stagnant, where prejudice overtook objectivity, where the science became irreversibly entangled with racism. How great the contrast between the ultimate course of genetics in Germany and the promise of international genetics displayed at the 1927 congress of genetics held in Berlin!

With the advent of Hitler, who himself had long advocated eugenic measures for race betterment, the eugenics movement in Germany became inextricably interwoven with the Nazi regime. Hitler's Minister of the Interior, Wilhelm Frick, proclaimed: "The fate of race-hygiene, of the Third Reich and the German people will in the future be indissolubly bound together."[102] Prominent eugenicists became Nazi officials, and Hitler filled his government with other men who at least sympathized with the eugenics program. Many of the private organizations concerned with eugenic education were reorganized as government agencies, the most prominent of which was the Kaiser Wilhelm Institute for Anthropology,

99. *Ibid.*, p. 20.
100. Baur, Fischer, and Lenz, *Human Heredity*, p. 677.
101. *Ibid.*, p. 5.
102. Cited by L. C. Dunn, "Cross Currents in the History of Human Genetics," *American Journal of Human Genetics*, 14(1962):8.

Human Genetics, and Eugenics, directed by Fischer. So strong was the institute's political affiliation with the Nazi state that it was not continued by the West German government after World War II.[103]

Human genetics and eugenics, distorted grotesquely for political ends, played a major role in determining the form of Nazi ideology.[104] Ideas of race and of Aryan superiority were fundamental components of Nazi culture, and Hitler's hopes of "national regeneration" rested upon what he considered the application of biological principles to human society. One German official remarked:

> The science of Heredity is by no means new. Its laws have been studied by many scientific associations and proclaimed before meetings. But it remained to one man to make the doctrine of heredity what it should be: *a state cause* (Staatsraison). This State Cause does not only concern Germany but all European peoples. But we may be the first to thank this *one* man, Adolf Hitler, and to follow him on the way towards a biological salvation of humanity.[105]

Fischer noted, "Everywhere the press is treating the questions of Race-Hygiene and Eugenics with the greatest interest, particularly since the Minister for propaganda, Dr. Goebbels, has done his utmost to spread ideas on heredity and biology. Race-Hygiene forms a substantial part of the national socialistic policy."[106] Although only a portion of the German geneticists who remained in the country accepted the Nazi and eugenic race doctrines, apparently even the bona fide scientists underestimated the dangers of the movement until it was too late.[107]

Such ideas received the force of law on July 14, 1933, when Hitler decreed the Hereditary Health Law, or Eugenic Sterilization Law, which was designed to ensure that "less worthy" members of the Third Reich did not pass on their genes. "Hereditary health courts," consisting of two state-appointed doctors and one state-appointed judge, decided whether a person was to be sterilized, with appeal to a "superior health court" possible. This law was not an innovation of the Nazis, for it had been preceded by thirty years of discussion of similar measures among German eugenicists; Germany quite possibly would have eventually established such a law without Hitler. However, unlike other countries with sterilization legisla-

103. *Ibid.*, p. 9.
104. For an excellent discussion of the literary, philosophical, and political origins of Nazi ideology, including racism, see Peter Viereck, *Meta-Politics: The Roots of the Nazi Mind* (New York: Capricorn Books, 1961).
105. "Eugenical Propaganda in Germany," *Eugenical News*, 19(1934):45.
106. "Eugenics in Germany," *Eugenical News*, 19(1934):43.
107. Dunn, "Cross Currents," p. 8.

tion, such as the United States, Finland, Sweden, Norway, Iceland, and the Canadian provinces of Alberta and British Columbia, Germany implemented its law immediately and on an enormous scale. During its first year of operation 56,244 persons deemed "hereditarily defective" by the eugenic courts were sterilized;[108] ultimately over 250,000 individuals underwent the operation.[109] This law began the process that led to experimentation with euthanasia, legalized by a decree of Hitler in 1939. Within two years 50,000 persons had been put to death under the euthanasia law—an experience which served as a useful laboratory for the eventual murder of millions of other "undesirables."[110]

"Eugenic" measures espoused by the Nazis were obviously a perversion of the true eugenic ideal as seen by well-meaning men deeply concerned about mankind's genetic future. Many individuals, both scientists and non-scientists, in the United States and across the world, pointed out that genuine eugenic ideology should not be confused with Nazi race doctrines. As the historian of medicine Henry Sigerist wrote, "I think it would be a great mistake to identify eugenic sterilization solely with the Nazi ideology and to dismiss the problem simply because we dislike the present German regime and its methods. . . . The [eugenic] problem is serious and acute, and we shall be forced to pay attention to it sooner or later."[111]

Such a distinction between "eugenic" and "Nazi" goals was not made by many leading American eugenicists, however. Most of them insisted, to quote Popenoe, that the Germans were "proceeding toward a policy that will accord with the best thought of eugenists in all civilized countries."[112] During the 1930's, a time when almost all American geneticists of standing viewed Germany's sterilization law with great suspicion, leading eugenicists in the United States praised the measure warmly, apparently not sensing the political motives which underlay the professed "eugenic" ones. The *Eugenical News* claimed: "It is difficult to see how the new German Sterilization Law could, as some have suggested, be deflected from its purely eugenical purpose, and be made an 'instrument of tyranny' for the sterilization of non-Nordic races."[113] A major defender of eugenic sterilization, Leon F. Whitney, wrote: "American Jewry is naturally suspecting that the

108. Samuel J. Holmes, *Human Genetics and its Social Import* (New York: McGraw-Hill Book Co., 1936), p. 374.

109. Henry E. Sigerist, *Civilization and Disease* (Ithaca, New York: Cornell University Press, 1943), p. 106.

110. Haller, *Eugenics*, p. 180; George L. Mosse, *Nazi Culture* (New York: Grosset and Dunlap, 1966), p. 60.

111. Sigerist, *Civilization and Disease*, pp. 106–7.

112. Popenoe, "German Sterilization Law," p. 260.

113. "Eugenical Sterilization in Germany," *Eugenical News*, 18(1933):90.

German chancellor had the law enacted for the specific purpose of steriliz-
ing the German Jews, but I believe nothing to be further from the
truth."[114] "The measure is solely eugenic in its purpose," he added, "and
were it not for its compulsory nature it would probably meet with the
approval of all who are free from religious bias."[115] In a letter to the
geneticist L. C. Dunn, Popenoe declared: "Not even Hitler proposes to
sterilize anyone on the ground of racial origin. My impression is that the
Germans are much more anxious to weed out the undesirable elements
among the Aryans, whatever these are, than to hit at any of the non-Aryan
groups."[116] He said also: "It remains to be seen whether sterilization in
Germany is more connected with politics than science. The law that has
been adopted is not a half-baked and hasty improvisation of the Hitler
regime, but is the product of many years of consideration by the best
specialists in Germany. . . . I must say that my impression is, from a careful following of the situation in the German scientific press, rather favorable."[117] Chided by Dunn for his apparently hasty endorsement of the
German measure, Popenoe replied: "I am surprised to hear that leading
geneticists in general do not support the eugenic program of sterilization. I
did not suppose there was any thoughtful geneticist who did not recognize
the desirability of sterilization under proper auspices, in selected cases."[118]

In the 1930's some American eugenicists began to sound more and
more like their German counterparts. Lothrop Stoddard described a Nazi
sterilization hearing and recorded his admiration for the German emphasis
upon biological fitness.[119] The reviewer of Grant's *Conquest of a Continent* for the *New York Times* wrote, "Substitute Aryan for Nordic, and a
good deal of Mr. Grant's argument would lend itself without much difficulty to the support of some recent pronouncements in Germany."[120]
Suspicions toward American eugenics did not diminish when Laughlin
received an honorary M.D. degree in 1936 from the University of Heidelberg.[121] Understandably, such developments alarmed most American ge-

114. Whitney, *The Case for Sterilization*, p. 138.
115. *Ibid.*, p. 138.
116. Paul Popenoe to L. C. Dunn, January 22, 1934, *LCD*.
117. *Ibid.*
118. *Ibid.*
119. Lothrop Stoddard, *Into the Darkness: Nazi Germany Today* (New York:
Duell, Sloan, & Pearce, 1940), pp. 179 ff.
120. New York *Times*, November 5, 1933, p. 16.
121. Ironically, prior to the 1930's the University of Heidelberg had been
reputed to be the furthest left of the German universities. Critics of Heidelberg often
would bemoan the large number of liberals on the staff. By 1932, however, Heidelberg had gone to the right, becoming the site of wild and emotional discussions of
racial problems. Addressing the medical faculty of Heidelberg one evening in 1932,

neticists and did much to convince them of the biases of most of the movement's enthusiasts. American and Nazi eugenics started to appear to them frighteningly alike.

Despite the American movement's surrender to racism, however, not all eugenic enthusiasts, even after World War I, were uncompromising villains; nor did eugenicists fail to make positive contributions to the science of genetics. As pointed out earlier, some eugenicists who were violently racist over the immigration question—most notably E. A. Ross—mellowed a decade later with the advent of fascism. Earlier still, between 1900 and 1915, when the newly rediscovered Mendelism was engaged in furious competition with biometry, the arguments of some of the scientifically oriented eugenicists such as Davenport and Castle helped demonstrate the universality of Mendelism, thereby contributing to the birth of the science of genetics. Nevertheless, eugenicists' clamoring ultimately proved to be their undoing. They exaggerated the power of heredity and belittled the role of environment long after that view was generally recognized to be incorrect. They tended to approach the subject of inheritance with a missionary zeal which made the cautious scientific geneticist highly uncomfortable. They enjoyed some immediate successes, but at the cost of ultimate failure.

geneticist Walter Landauer, who had studied zoology and genetics at Heidelberg in the early 1920's, noted this transition in his alma mater. Competing with him that night was a very emotional and well-attended mass meeting on "the race question." (Conversation with Walter Landauer, January 26, 1971.)

6

Repudiation of Eugenics

After World War I, as the eugenics movement in America acquired more and more of a racist tone, many prominent geneticists became increasingly doubtful of it. Their distrust began while they witnessed the movement's role in the passage of the Immigration Restriction Act; their suspicions heightened in the 1930's as they observed eugenics in America to be similar to eugenics in Germany. No longer tolerant of the movement's inadequacies, many American geneticists publicly began to condemn it. Some geneticists had pointed out the weaknesses of the eugenics program even before America's entry into the first World War, but these earlier criticisms tended to be mild and usually did not question the ethics or motives of the eugenicists. After the mid-1920's geneticists issued much harsher pronouncements which they hoped the public as well as their colleagues would heed. Not all geneticists shared the same degree of hostility toward eugenics, of course. Some, including Morgan, Pearl, and Jennings, severed any affiliation with the movement they might once have had; others, most notably East, Conklin, and Holmes, remained at least nominal eugenicists and to the end participated occasionally in the movement's activities. But among all these men, even those who remained to some degree personally involved with the movement, a fundamental change in attitude had occurred. Their pre-war enthusiasm and their war-time realization of the impediments to eugenic programs had both disappeared, to be replaced by a feeling of deep concern regarding the motives of the movement's racist leadership.

During the period immediately following World War I, a few geneticists first began to express dismay at many eugenicists' subjugation of genetic theories to political purposes. In an article in *Scribner's Magazine* in 1919, Conklin debunked much of the racial discussion then proceeding in America. He did not mention the eugenics movement directly by name, but he did express his unhappiness that "racial, varietal, national, and class antagonisms have arisen everywhere, and have often led to terrible hostilities."[1] He felt that racial enmity was unjustified for biological as well as for humanitarian reasons. "Biology shows that we are all cousins if not brothers [because of common lines of ancestry]," he wrote. "As a result of this common descent human resemblances are vastly more numerous and important than the differences."[2] He also indicated that differences among the various European stocks, from which most Americans were descended, are very slight, thereby ridiculing the current debate as to which of these stocks are the "fitter" and should be preferentially admitted as immigrants to the country. "The inherent antagonisms between these stocks that agitators and designing politicians tell us about are really not inherent at all," he declared, "but are largely created, cultivated, and magnified by education and environment for national and selfish purposes."[3] With similar intent, Holmes pointed out in 1923:

There is an extensive literature on race mixture, but from the scientific standpoint most of it is exceedingly superficial and disappointing. It is frequently marred by prejudice, and rarely is any attempt made to separate the social and the biological factors that conspire to determine the status and characteristics of mixed breeds. Both those who favor and those who oppose the mixture of races appeal to the results of crossing varieties of plants and animals in support of their position, and succeed in finding biological analogies of the desired kind.[4]

Despite such pleas, the eugenices movement became more and more involved with questions of race.

Until the mid-1920's, few geneticists made public statements like those of Conklin and Holmes. Most investigators were preoccupied with their experiments, not expecting the movement to be a significant political force. With the impending passage of the Immigration Restriction Act, however, many geneticists began to view the eugenics movement with much greater unhappiness than before. Alarmed by eugenicists' distortions of genetics, they realized that they could no longer countenance its activities. For years they had been losing interest in the movement; now they began to denounce it. In late 1923 and early 1924 several noted geneticists—among them H. S. Jennings, R. Pearl, Vernon Kellogg, E. Carlton MacDowell, and Samuel J. Holmes—began correspondence over

1. E. G. Conklin, "Biology and Democracy," *Scribner's Magazine*, 65(1919):408.
2. *Ibid.*, pp. 407–8.
3. *Ibid.*, p. 408.
4. Samuel J. Holmes, *Studies in Evolution and Eugenics* (New York: Harcourt, Brace and Company, 1923), p. 218.

the immigration issue, expressing the common fear that selective restrictive legislation might pass.[5] They were not necessarily against the idea of restricting immigration since they realized that this could be one means of combating overpopulation in the country. Nevertheless, they objected to the pending legislation because they felt it was based on prejudice rather than science. As the movement's outpouring of propaganda increased, many workers began to put their feelings into print. Though they were taken too much by surprise to influence the outcome of the immigration bill, they nevertheless helped bring about the movement's demise.

One of the first to utter such protests was Jennings, an outstanding protozoan geneticist who after World War I had become one of America's foremost expositors of applying only sound biology to human affairs. On many occasions during the next several years he publicly spoke out against the excesses of the eugenics movement in order to expose the false biology at its base. In the December 15, 1923, issue of *The Survey*, examining the same data used by Laughlin in his report to Congress, he demonstrated that "it does not appear to be established that the recent immigrants are inferior in their inherited qualities."[6] He expressed the hope that his re-analysis of the data would "discourage attempts to regulate immigration on the basis of race and nationality, so far as Europeans are concerned."[7] A few months later, writing in *Science*, he again pointed out that "on the basis of Laughlin's findings a European-born population constituted as in 1890 would contribute practically exactly the same number of institutional defectives as an equal European-born population constituted as in 1910."[8] In *Prometheus* (1925) he severely criticized eugenicists for spreading a doctrine based upon outmoded principles of biology. He stated: "Knowledge has moved rapidly and has, indeed, changed fundamentally within the last ten years, altering the picture as to the relations of heredity and environment. What has gotten into popular consciousness as Mendelism—still presented in the conventional biological gospels—has become grotesquely inadequate and misleading."[9] He particularly deplored the use of such principles to justify racist propaganda on immigration,

5. For example, see Raymond Pearl to Herbert Jennings, November 24, 1923; Samuel J. Holmes to Jennings, January 30, 1924; Jennings to Holmes, February 5, 1924; Holmes to Jennings, January 29, 1924; Jennings to Vernon Kellogg, February 14, 1924; E. Carleton MacDowell to Jennings, February 20, 1924; all *HSJ.*
6. Herbert S. Jennings, "Undesirable Aliens," *The Survey*, 51(1923):311.
7. *Ibid.*, p. 364.
8. Herbert S. Jennings, "Proportion of Defectives from the Northwest and from the Southeast of Europe," *Science*, N. S., 59(1924):256.
9. Herbert S. Jennings, *Prometheus* (New York: E. P. Dutton and Co., 1925), p. 11.

claiming that eugenicists held a "perfectly empty and idle view of the matter."[10] In the *Encyclopedia of the Social Sciences* in 1930 he had some of his harshest words yet for the eugenics movement:

> National and racial prejudices have entered largely into eugenic propaganda. One of the commonest objectives has been the maintenance of the purity or the dominance of a certain racial or national group—the group selected for preference being that to which the selectors belong. This factor has entered largely into the eugenic agitation for restriction of immigration. Both racial arrogance and the desire to justify present social systems find a congenial field in eugenic propaganda.[11]

Other geneticists in the mid-1920's also joined the attack. In the preface to *Mankind at the Crossroads* (1924), East contended that eugenicists have shown "too great a tendency to push ahead of the facts."[12] "Eugenics," he wrote, "a one-sided ill-considered eugenics, has been a veritable honey-pot for the dilettante and the amateur. They have buzzed around, circulating propaganda of a singularly pernicious type, plausible fallacies alleged to have a scientific background."[13] The following year, in *Evolution and Genetics*, Morgan complained of "the somewhat acrimonious discussion taking place at the present time concerning racial differences in man."[14] In the last chapter, not present in the first edition of the book in 1917, he examined the issue of hereditary differences among races, pointing out that "all the races of mankind have an enormous number of genes in common and only a few that are different. The latter produces the relatively slight structural differences that are found in different races."[15] "A little good will," he added, "might seem more fitting in these complicated questions than the attitude adopted by some of the modern race-propagandists."[16] In 1926, writing in the *Encyclopedia Britannica* on the subject of eugenics, Castle deplored the movement's lack of a legitimate scientific foundation. "A considerable portion of the published material [on eugenics]," he stated, "is probably of small value, since it is uncontrolled by experiment and is based largely on uncritical data."[17] The next

10. *Ibid.*, p. 66.
11. Herbert S. Jennings, "Eugenics," in *The Encyclopaedia of the Social Sciences*, 1st ed. (1930), p. 621.
12. Edward M. East, *Mankind at the Crossroads* (New York: Charles Scribner's Sons, 1924), p. vi.
13. *Ibid.*, p. vi.
14. T. H. Morgan, *Evolution and Genetics*, rev. ed. (Princeton: Princeton University Press, 1925), p. vi.
15. *Ibid.*, p. 184.
16. *Ibid.*, p. 207.
17. William E. Castle, "Eugenics," *Encyclopedia Britannica*, 13th ed. (1926), p. 1031.

year, in an article in *The American Mercury*, Pearl expressed his irritation with the misleading scientific statements eugenicists had been making to justify their programs. "In preaching as they do," he wrote, "that like produces like, and that therefore superior people will have superior children, and inferior people inferior children, the orthodox eugenicists are going contrary to the best established facts of genetical science, and are, in the long run, doing their cause harm."[18] Pearl, whose enthusiasm for eugenics before the war had seemingly been boundless, was now of the view that "it would seem to be high time that eugenics cleaned house, and threw away the old-fashioned rubbish which has accumulated in the attic."[19]

Thus, dismayed at eugenicists' distortion of their science to justify their political goals—in particular, selective immigration restriction—many prominent geneticists in the middle and late 1920's began to condemn the movement. It is understandable that they became so greatly embittered. The racial hostility engendered by the movement ran counter to many geneticists' humanistic values and strong feelings of compassion and understanding for their fellow man. Jennings, for example, considered by some of his friends to be a "sentimental humanitarian," was of the view that "good will toward men" should be the vision of excellence in a society with eugenic goals.[20] Moreover, eugenicists' biased interpretations of genetic findings were incompatible with geneticists' view of the importance of critically and objectively evaluating scientific evidence, regardless of the conclusions favored. As Castle told Davenport: "Of course you don't expect me, in matters scientific to accept *any* view except as I am convinced of the soundness of the evidence on which it rests. One can't trust even his own *views*, much less another's. We want incontrovertible facts, no matter whose views they favor."[21] Thus, eugenicists offended both geneticists' sense of human values and their conception of legitimate scientific research. Geneticists accordingly spoke out against the movement for social and political as well as for scientific reasons. In this light their strong reaction against it can be best understood.

The 1930's witnessed the culmination of geneticists' revulsion against the eugenics movement. In that decade the genetic argument against eugenic proposals became fully mature. The work of Lionel Penrose, an

18. Raymond Pearl, "The Biology of Superiority," *The American Mercury*, 12(1927):266.
19. *Ibid.*, p. 266.
20. A letter from the *Independent Woman* magazine to Herbert S. Jennings, February 9, 1934, *HSJ*. The magazine in this letter had sent Jennings a questionnaire; the above quote is a reply he had written on it in pencil.
21. W. E. Castle to C. B. Davenport, March 19, 1918, *CBD*.

English physician and geneticist, and others showed that feeble-mindedness, contrary to the claims of many eugenicists, was not a uniform disease entity determined by a single recessive gene but a condition which could arise from a variety of complex causes. The rapid elimination of feeblemindedness from the population by sterilization had been a singular proposal of eugenicists; now that the condition was seen to have such a complex etiology, their simple solution to the problem could not be so facilely justified. The growth of population genetics in the 1920's and early 1930's carried with it perhaps the most biting of all intellectual criticisms of eugenic programs: the demonstration that, even granting eugenicists their assumptions of the omnipotence of heredity and the Mendelian recessive mode of inheritance of many traits, a program of "positive" and "negative" eugenics would not bring about the rapid improvement in the genetic quality of the people that eugenicists had claimed. Population genetics was concerned with changes in gene frequencies in human populations; various writers had determined the mathematical consequences of selection of different intensities on cross-breeding populations. One important conclusion was that changes in gene frequencies resulting from selection against recessive traits would occur too slowly to be of practical use for a eugenics program.[22]

In addition to these developments in genetics, the attack on eugenicists' racial notions had been bolstered by arguments from other disciplines. By the 1930's the work of Franz Boas and some of his students, among them Ruth Benedict and Margaret Mead, had revolutionized anthropology. Boas had rebelled against the conventional anthropological approach of judging the ideas and institutions of non-Western cultures, particularly primitive peoples, by the standards of our own society. Recognizing that culture reflects a people's social and historical experiences, he also had rejected the widely held assumption that every race or society represents some stage on a linear scale of progression from lower to higher. In the 1920's he and other anthropologists denounced the ideas of Grant, Stoddard, and Osborn; in the 1930's these anthropologists vehemently protested the racial theories of Nazi propagandists. Many psychologists had begun to recognize that a person's performance on intelligence tests is determined in part by his training, background, and culture; some who had formerly

22. L. C. Dunn has suggested that one reason men like Conklin, East, and Holmes continued as cautious, non-racist eugenicists in the 1920's and 1930's was that they never had worked out the mathematical consequences of selection on gene frequencies. They were critical experimentalists, but, Conklin and Holmes at least, unfamiliar and uncomfortable with the theoretical work proceeding in population genetics. (Conversation with L. C. Dunn, October 15, 1970.)

argued for a racial scale of intelligence began to reverse themselves. C. C. Brigham, who in 1923 had claimed that the army IQ tests reaffirmed Madison Grant's idea that Nordics were mentally superior to Alpines and Mediterraneans, by 1930 had changed his mind. "Comparative studies of various national and racial groups may not be made with existing tests," he admitted. "In particular one of the most pretentious of these comparative racial studies—the writer's own—was without foundation."[23] Such writers were not necessarily trying to demonstrate intellectual equality among races but were pointing to the difficulties in differentiating hereditary from environmental influences in determining a person's IQ score. (By the 1930's, however, environmentalist explanations of human nature, Marxism, Freudianism, and behaviorism, were also in vogue.) Taken together, these arguments refuted virtually the entirety of eugenicists' scientific views. Eugenic proposals could be shown to be untenable without them, but these criticisms added considerable fuel to the fire.

In the 1930's many geneticists' distrust of racism and eugenics increased further as social conditions changed. The Great Depression punished economically the Nordic and non-Nordic alike; individuals who had lost their incomes could no longer convincingly argue that wealth and social standing are measures of genetic fitness. More important, the Nazis espoused a creed of Aryan purity and superiority and a morbid fascination with health, biological fitness, and human breeding. Geneticists' response to the German situation evidently began in earnest in the spring of 1933 after three thousand German scholars were dismissed from their posts for racial or political reasons. Initially some American geneticists had not thought that their dismissal would be permanent. Pearl remarked: "I have a strong feeling that the present attitude of the German administration regarding such men will be only temporary, and that as a matter of fact most such men will gravitate back to their old positions within a year at most."[24] However, such optimism soon vanished; most geneticists quickly began to realize that Hitler had no intention of revoking his proclamation. L. C. Dunn, a mammalian geneticist at Columbia University, wrote: "Apparently the 'responsible' heads of the government have recognized this error in regard to the Jewish question and would gladly find a way out which would rescind it all and yet save their faces. . . . This is a belief expressed to me by a few others, but in my judgment, it is a Freudian wish."[25] A few months later, following Hitler's enactment of the "eu-

23. C. C. Brigham, "Intelligence Tests of Immigrant Groups," *Psychological Review*, 37(1930):165.
24. Raymond Pearl to L. C. Dunn, May 24, 1933, *LCD.*
25. L. C. Dunn to Alfred Cohn, June 20, 1933, *LCD.*

genic" sterilization measure, geneticists' distrust of the German regime became greater still. Dunn wrote:

> The business of finding out the characteristics of the German population goes on vigorously. I saw in Munich the new census sheets which everyone must fill out. The information wanted was clearly designed to "place" everyone so that the authorities would know where they stood racially and politically. From our point of view I see no way out. At close range, the situation is heart-breaking.[26]

Muller complained: "Genetics has been very much perverted by the Fascists. Their perverted version, with its emphasis on human race-differences, is used by them as an important part of the theoretical basis of the whole Fascist ideology, in the name of which so many atrocities are committed."[27] "Suffice it to say," he pointed out, "that there is not one iota of evidence from genetics for any such conclusions, and it is too bad to have them issued with the apparent stamp of genetic authority. They form just the sort of ground which reactionaries desire, on which to raise a pseudoscientific edifice for the defense of their system of sex, class and race exploitation."[28]

As geneticists became distrustful of the Nazis, they became more and more hostile toward the American eugenics movement. They had good reason to view the American movement with apprehension, since many American eugenicists had been forthright in their praise of Nazi "eugenic" measures. Fearing that what was happening in Germany might happen in America, many geneticists found their unhappiness with the eugenics movement reaching a climax. To emphasize this important point, it is worth quoting Dunn in detail:

> With genetics its [eugenics'] relations have always been close, although there have been distinct signs of cleavage in recent years, chiefly due to the feeling on the part of many geneticists that eugenic research was not always activated by purely disinterested scientific motives, but was influenced by social and political considerations tending to bring about too rapid application of incompletely proved theses. . . .
> I have just observed in Germany some of the consequences of reversing the order as between program and discovery. The incomplete knowledge of today, much of it based on a theory of the state which has been influenced by the racial, class, and religious prejudices of the group in power, has been embalmed in law, and the avenues to improvement in the techniques of improving the population have been completely closed. Al-

26. *Ibid.*
27. H. J. Muller, "Genetics and Society," *Fact* (London), 27(June, 1939):92.
28. H. J. Muller, "Human Heredity," *Birth Control Review*, 17(1933):21.

though some progress may be made in reducing the proportion of those elements which are undesirable to the regime, the cost appears to be tremendous. The genealogical record offices have become powerful agencies of the state, and medical judgments even when possible, appear to be subservient to political purposes. Apart from the injustices in individual cases, and the loss of personal liberty, the solution of the whole eugenic problem by fiat eliminates any rational solution by free competition of ideas and evidence. Scientific progress in general seems to have a very dark future. Altho much of this is due to the dictatorship, it seems to illustrate the dangers which all programs run which are not continually responsive to new knowledge, and should certainly strengthen the resolve which we generally have in the U.S. to keep all agencies which contribute to such questions as free as possible from commitment to fixed programs.[29]

In the 1930's geneticists' repudiation of the movement took many forms. Some, such as Dunn and Muller, spoke out individually against the movement. The dismay of many geneticists with the German situation helped instigate a shake-up in the editorial policies of the *Journal of Heredity*, which until then had been publishing many uncritical articles favorable toward eugenics. Throughout the 1930's, numerous geneticists— including Curt Stern, A. F. Shull, A. F. Blakeslee, R. A. Emerson, C. H. Danforth, L. C. Dunn, Laurence Snyder, Sewall Wright, Barbara McClintock, Raymond Pearl, and L. J. Cole—worked for the American Committee for Displaced German Scholars, an organization which attempted to relocate displaced German academicians in American institutions.[30] In 1939 a group of geneticists at the Seventh International Genetics Congress at Edinburgh issued a widely publicized condemnation of eugenics, racism, and Nazi doctrines.[31] Not all geneticists could take time off from the laboratory to speak out against the eugenics movement, but those who did expressed views held generally by geneticists. For example, Walter Landauer, a geneticist at the University of Connecticut, was not an outspoken public figure on the matter; nevertheless, like most geneticists, he also found the views of American and Nazi eugenicists to be

29. L. C. Dunn to John Merriam, July 3, 1935, *LCD*.
30. The Dunn Papers provide a poignant account of the human problems involved in the relocation of displaced German scholars. The Committee had to balance its humanitarian goal of aiding the refugees with the practical consideration of how not to stifle American scholarship by offering positions to Germans rather than to young Americans. The Committee's usual compromise was to try to find positions for refugees which otherwise would not have been filled. This compromise was often emotionally trying for the refugees, however, since many men who had been leading scholars in Germany had to accept obscure, unimportant positions in America.
31. The "manifesto" may be found in "Men and Mice at Edinburgh: Reports from the Genetics Congress," *Journal of Heredity*, 30(1939):371–74.

distasteful. Though he wrote little on the issue, he frequently pointed out the flaws in eugenic reasoning in lectures and conversations.[32]

While they were renouncing the eugenics movement in the 1930's, some geneticists for the first time manifested a sense of "social responsibility" in its modern form. It is again worth quoting Dunn in detail:

The effects of this knowledge [genetic science] upon society have been quite different in different countries. The demonstration that certain differences between individuals are influenced by heredity and hence by ancestry has led in Germany to the promulgation and enforcement of laws requiring the elimination of persons with certain characteristics from the breeding population. If you live in Germany you can be hauled before a court and sentenced to be sterilized for any one of a number of offenses committed when you chose your ancestors. . . .

In our own country the immigration quotas were set some time ago after hearings at which alleged mental differences between European races, presumably of a genetic and therefore permanent character, played a large part in determining a policy which has guided our democracy for twenty years.

What can science do for democracy? It can tell the people the truth about such misuses of the prestige of science; the facts in these cases did not matter—they were opposed to the practice which resulted, but not enough people knew them well enough or lacked the courage to make them known.

Since the people have come to accept pronouncements made in the name of science, chiefly I think because of the prestige gained through material and technological advances made possible through science, it behooves scientists to be aware of the responsibility which this trust and support implies.[33]

Dunn's speech clearly represents an explicit statement of what is today sometimes referred to as the scientist's social responsibility: his duty to inform the public of the scientific facts of a public question concerning the application of science or technology to social problems so that an enlightened citizenry may more knowledgeably make important political, ethical, or social decisions. The term implies something other than the mere participation of a scientist in politics. From this perspective, a scientist lobbying in Congress for partisan purposes, such as increased federal support of scientific research, would not necessarily be exercising social responsibility. Neither would a scientist expressing his views on general political issues, such as the Vietnamese War. The term also suggests a

32. Conversation with Walter Landauer, January 26, 1971.
33. L. C. Dunn, "Natural Science and Democracy," copy of radio address delivered on Armistice Day, 1937, LCD.

necessary distinction between an investigator's role as scientist and as citizen. A scientist has human limitations; in exercising social responsibility properly he must make no pretense of possessing greater *moral* insight into the beneficial use of science than the non-scientist. Many investigators have personal views as to how science should be used, but these are their views as "citizens," not as "scientists." Social responsibility demands the analysis and elucidation of scientific knowledge, not the prescription of social policy.

Geneticists' sense of social responsibility appears to have developed in response to the misuse of the science of genetics in America and Germany. This fact suggests a general explanation for understanding why certain groups of scientists have developed social responsibility—namely, social responsibility results from a *crisis* in the social uses of science. In the case of geneticists, this crisis was the use of genetic theory to justify immigration restriction in the United States and sterilization programs in Nazi Germany. This crisis wrought such tragic consequences that geneticists began to conceive it as their *responsibility* to guard against any further perversions of their science.

In modern times, it appears that every group of scientists which has developed a sense of social responsibility has done so following a crisis in the social uses of their science. The example of physicists is obvious; the social impact of the atomic bomb was so great that many of them began to conceive it as their duty to explain atomic energy to interested congressmen and laymen. With the founding of the *Bulletin of the Atomic Scientists* in 1945, physicists made a moral commitment to this purpose which remains with them today. Biochemists and chemists concerned with the use of chemical weapons also developed their concern after a crisis, the use of chemical weapons by the United States government on civilian populations. In the spring of 1967 they led five thousand American scientists in petitioning President Johnson to end production of these arms. By leading discussions of the ethical implications of medical research, physicians also have shown social responsibility. They most effectively have fulfilled this responsibility during certain "crises" in the history of medicine, such as the employment of the diphtheria and tetanus anti-toxins in the late nineteenth century and the bold experimentation in transplanting human organs in the 1960's.

On first glance, it appears that geneticists' harsh repudiation of the eugenics movement contradicts the widely held notion of the "utilitarian aspect" of scientific discovery. If it is assumed that scientists are greatly influenced by the demands of society, the failure of geneticists in the 1920's to support the Immigration Restriction Act in large numbers is difficult to explain. Why did they not direct their own research to see if they could "prove" the validity and justness of that very popular law? The answer to this question is inherent in the observation that whenever science and society interact, science, if it is to remain science, above all must maintain its *autonomy*. By "autonomy" is meant not an external independence and detachment from the social fabric—indeed, one of the premises of this book is that this type of independence does not exist—but rather the ability of science to maintain its internal standards of truth. It must be remembered that "the standard of truth in science has nothing to do with the criteria of political success or of political loyalty. A scientific proposition is true or false in accordance with the standards which are appropriate to scientific judgment."[34] The political subjugation of a science certainly jeopardizes the possibility of objective investigation. Though the "utilitarian bias" indeed influences how a science is applied, that science, if it is to survive, must be committed to scientific truth, not to the justification of a political viewpoint.

Geneticists' development of social responsibility in the late 1920's and 1930's may be interpreted in effect as an assertion by these men of the internal autonomy of their discipline; what has earlier been called a "crisis" may also be viewed as a threat to the intellectual autonomy of the science. In challenging the eugenics movement, geneticists disputed its scientific and moral merits without stating explicitly that they were "defending the autonomy of genetics." Still, the end result was the same as if they had, since a compromise with legitimate standards of proof and methodology might have marked the end of their science's autonomy.

Thus, though many geneticists had been losing interest in the eugenics movement since the beginning of World War I, after the war their disillusionment with the movement entered a second phase, a stage characterized by their public repudiation of the movement. Underlying their condemnations was a deep aversion to the movement's subjugation of genetic principles to justify preconceived social and political ideologies. In the 1920's geneticists protested the movement's use of genetic theory to justify selective immigration restriction legislation; in the 1930's they feared its similarities with eugenics in Nazi Germany. The second stage of geneticists' withdrawal from the movement was therefore prompted mainly by social rather than intellectual events. These events constituted a crisis in the social use of genetics. By developing a sense of social responsibility, many

---

34. Edward A. Shils, "The Autonomy of Science," in Bernard Barber and Walter Hirsch, eds., *Sociology of Science* (New York: The Free Press of Glencoe, 1962), p. 611.

workers in the field took part in the resolution of this crisis. Geneticists, who before the war had helped to establish the movement, now helped to destroy it.

The geneticists usually spoke out against the movement as individuals and not as groups. The Genetics Society of America, for example, did not prepare a formal condemnation of eugenic or Nazi race doctrines in the 1930's despite considerable discussion at its annual meetings about doing so. Scientific organizations are often reluctant to dispense the edicts of "science." Moreover, there seems to be a tendency for scientists to speak on social issues in their own name; scientists frequently dislike being spoken for. This was the case with the Genetics Society; its members could not be persuaded to go on record as a society.[35] The best-known group statement by geneticists against race doctrines was that issued at the Seventh International Congress of Genetics at Edinburgh in 1939—the so-called "Geneticists' Manifesto"—but this was actually a resolution informally circulated among certain of the participants and not a formal statement by the congress.

In criticizing the movement's racism, geneticists were not claiming that all races are equal. Indeed, in 1932 even so ardent a foe of eugenic and Nazi race doctrines as the English biologist J. B. S. Haldane wrote a book entitled *The Inequality of Man.* Rather, they were urging that no man or race be unfairly judged. They pointed to the difficulties in differentiating environmental from hereditary influences in human development, and they expressed the view that no one race has a monopoly on desirable qualities. "One can assert that deaf-mutism is commoner among Jews than among Gentiles without incurring the charge of anti-Semitism,"[36] wrote the English geneticist Lancelot Hogben. "With so many diagnosable physical ailments to choose from," he added, "it is possible for normal people to discuss the occupational or racial distribution of any single disease of the body without assuming a tone of impudent superiority."[37] Moreover, most geneticists did not renounce the eugenic ideal of working for the genetic improvement of mankind. As Jennings wrote in 1931: "In spite of the difficulties and aberrations the better considered aims of eugenics . . . may be held as desirable and their realization to some degree not out of the range of possibility."[38] Nevertheless, so many eugenic

35. Conversation with L. C. Dunn, October 15, 1970. Dunn was the first president of the Genetics Society, which had been organized in 1932.

36. Lancelot Hogben, *Nature and Nurture*, rev. ed. (New York: W. W. Norton and Company, 1939), p. 31.

37. *Ibid.*, p. 31.

38. Jennings, "Eugenics," p. 621.

devotees displayed such brazen indifference to truth that many geneticists became greatly discouraged over the prospects that anyone could ever approach the matter objectively and cautiously. To some geneticists this was a cause of bitter disappointment. They objected to the eugenics movement in practice, not in principle.

7
Inhibition of Human Genetics

1. The Decline of Human Genetics

In the 1930's research in human genetics in the United States nearly came to a standstill. A major reason for this was the difficulty that the discipline faced overcoming numerous technical impediments. However, the field was hindered additionally by its close association with the eugenics movement. From the start, investigation in human genetics had been dominated by eugenic devotees who were more strongly committed to dubious social and political causes than to sound scientific method. In the mid-1920's, while the eugenicists were quoting much unscientific literature on race and class genetics to justify selective immigration restriction, many geneticists began expressing dissatisfaction with the field. In the 1930's their dissatisfaction turned into dismay as they witnessed Hitler's rise to power. They criticized research in human genetics for both scientific and social-ethical reasons: they objected to the carelessness and superficiality of much of the work in the field as well as to the hasty and premature utilization of the results of such studies to support distasteful political doctrines. Some geneticists had voiced unhappiness with the field before this time, but after the mid-1920's they criticized it much more harshly. (David Heron's previously cited evaluation of human genetics was unusually severe compared to others written before the mid-1920's.) Their criticisms of research in human genetics cannot be entirely separated from the public attacks on the eugenics movement which they were making simultaneously; their disillusionment with the latter helped bring disrepute upon the former. This was almost inevitable because the two activities were so closely associated. These criticisms showed that the domination of human genetics by eugenicists was indeed detrimental to the science. Among most geneticists there grew such a suspicion that human genetics would be used only for political purposes that many who once might have contributed to the field now refused to do so.

The inhibitory effect that eugenics had upon human genetics could be seen in many ways. During the late 1920's and 1930's, several institutions devoted to promoting research in the inheritance of man either terminated their association with the eugenics movement or faded away. For example, the Minnesota Eugenics Society, founded in 1922 with the funds and leadership of Dr. Charles Fremont Dight, quickly achieved a degree of influence but by 1930 had dissolved. The society was revived in 1945 as the Minnesota Human Genetics League, an organization devoted primarily to pure research rather than to eugenic applications. None of the forty-seven charter members of the league was a holdover from the earlier eugenics society.[1] Dight similarly bequested funds for the Dight Institute for the Promotion of Human Genetics, founded in 1941 and first directed by Clarence P. Oliver, a radiation geneticist now at the University of Texas. The institute at first had to overcome the suspicion of many people that studies in human heredity were merely a sideline for eugenics. One physician initially refused to help Oliver with the institute but later changed his mind after he saw that the institute was indeed pursuing human genetics for academic and not eugenic purposes.[2]

Similarly, many journals which had been publishing studies on human heredity disappeared, and those which continued to operate terminated their affiliation with eugenics. The most notable example was the *Journal of Heredity*. From its start the journal had published many uncritical articles on human inheritance and eugenics, but in the early 1930's the dismay of a group of influential geneticists with eugenics prompted a re-examination of the journal's editorial policies. Dunn confided to Castle: "At present the journal is a hodge-podge—partly scientific report, partly newspaper, partly popular science and occasionally propaganda. I should like to see it serve its purpose better."[3] Castle replied, "I don't care for some of the eugenics articles, should be glad indeed to have the Journal keep out of that field altogether."[4] Prompted by such prominent investigators, the journal in the mid-1930's drastically altered its policies toward these subjects. An editorial in 1939 announced the completion of these policy changes:

1. Sheldon C. Reed, "The Local Eugenics Society," *The American Journal of Human Genetics*, 9(1957):1.
2. Clarence P. Oliver to author, August 4, 1970.
3. L. C. Dunn to William E. Castle, March 14, 1933, *LCD*.
4. W. E. Castle to L. C. Dunn, March 20, 1933, *LCD*.

We have had some discussion in the Journal in the past few years of possible planks for eugenic platforms. It is felt that developments in eugenic thought, both here and abroad, have in recent years reached a point where a complete and critical re-evaluation of eugenic philosophy and of proposals for action is necessary if the eugenic point of view is to have any place in directing human biological and social conservation and evolution.[5]

Accordingly the journal dropped the name "eugenics" from its subtitle and ceased publishing biased investigations relating to man.[6]

Other publications also revised their positions toward work in human genetics. For five years after its formation by William Bateson and R. C. Punnett in 1910, the *Journal of Genetics* regularly published articles on human inheritance. All of these papers consisted of pedigree analyses, and some suffered greatly from uncritical preparation and interpretation. One study attempted to show that the "peculiar facial expression recognised as Jewish" followed a simple Mendelian pattern of inheritance, and another tried to prove that musical sense and artistic ability are Mendelian recessives.[7] The last paper of this sort appeared in 1916; for fourteen years thereafter the *Journal* published no material at all on human genetics. Only in the 1930's did articles on the subject reappear in the *Journal*, and these consisted of sophisticated statistical treatments of the problems of human inheritance. The *Annals of Eugenics*, under the editorship of Lionel Penrose, belatedly changed its name in 1954 to the *Annals of Human Genetics*. Penrose had never liked the association between eugenics and human genetics and wanted to make this change in 1946 when he became editor, but R. A. Fisher, who had preceded him in that position, opposed it. Far from being a zealous eugenicist, Fisher in fact regarded the members of the Eugenics Education Society as stupid. He had even incurred the enmity of the Society by using a grant from it for his own researches rather than for eugenic investigations as it had intended. He agreed with

5. Editor, "A Quarterly Eugenics Section," *Journal of Heredity*, 30(1939):108.
6. As mentioned earlier, even before the end of the first World War some geneticists disagreed with the *Journal of Heredity*'s editorial policy on matters of eugenics and human heredity. The moment was not yet ripe for the *Journal* to revise its policy on these subjects, however. A delay was necessary for new editorial leadership to emerge, for additional developments within genetics to cast eugenicists' scientific assumptions even more in doubt, and for the climate of the Depression years to discredit eugenicists' social and ethical views. (Conversation with Sewall Wright, September 24, 1970.)
7. Redcliffe N. Salaman, "Heredity and the Jew," *Journal of Genetics*, 1(1911):276; H. Drinkwater, "Inheritance of Artistic and Mental Ability," *Journal of Genetics*, 5(1916):229.

eugenics in principle, however, and felt that certain steps might properly be taken, such as family allowances graded in proportion to income. He considered changing the journal's title tantamount to taking away the flag of a ship. Despite Fisher's objections, Penrose eventually accomplished the change.[8] Even textbooks which entered multiple editions abandoned their earlier orientation toward eugenics. R. Ruggles Gates admitted that he was motivated to write *Heredity and Eugenics* in 1923 "by my interest in Eugenics."[9] That edition of the book included a fifty-page chapter entitled "Social and World Aspects of Eugenics" as well as many briefer discussions of eugenic problems. Subsequent editions in 1930 and 1946 dropped the term "eugenics" from the book and chapter titles. Though these editions did contain extended discussions of racial crossing, an item of paramount interest to eugenicists, they seldom referred to eugenics by name. To see these changes in a book by Gates was especially remarkable since many biologists of the day considered him a racist and his views biased and inaccurate.[10]

Not only established periodicals viewed human genetics with increased caution; so also did many newly organized journals. Two of the most notable of these were the *Quarterly Review of Biology* and *Human Biology*, both founded in the late 1920's by Raymond Pearl. During the first

8. Conversations with Lionel Penrose, January 25 and 26, 1971. Also, conversation with Harry Harris, December 16, 1970.

9. R. Ruggles Gates, *Heredity and Eugenics* (New York: Macmillan Co., 1923), p. vii.

10. As a cytologist Gates performed admirable work, and some consider him rather than Calvin Bridges to be the discoverer of non-disjunction (failure of a pair of chromosomes to separate at meiosis). However, his studies of human genetics contained careless thinking intermixed with critical reasoning. He once pointed out that a study which had concluded that immigrants have a higher percentage of feeble-mindedness than native-born Americans did not remember "that a trans-Atlantic voyage under steerage conditions is not a very good preparation for such a [IQ] test," but he also felt that non-white races are more primitive than Caucasians and as late as 1949 he quoted a pre-World War I study by Davenport which allegedly showed that the tendency to violent temper is a Mendelian dominant trait. Many biologists of the day considered him a racist or at best racist-influenced. Haldane objected to a paper he had written for the *Eugenics Review* on the grounds that it "ranks itself as a propagandist rather than a scientific work." Haldane added: "If statements of this kind are used to support the eugenics movement a certain number of scientific students of heredity are likely to hold aloof from it."

In recent letters to the author both C. P. Oliver and Lionel Penrose commented on Gates' reputation among his contemporaries.

R. Ruggles Gates, *Heredity in Man* (New York: The Macmillan Company, 1930), pp. 334, 335; R. Ruggles Gates, *Pedigrees of Negro Families* (Philadelphia: The Blakiston Company, 1949), p. 160; J. B. S. Haldane, "Letter to the Editor," *Eugenics Review*, 28(1937):333; Clarence P. Oliver to author, August 4, 1970; Lionel S. Penrose to author, October 13, 1970.

decade of the century, when the eugenics movement was getting underway in America, Pearl was unreserved in his support of the movement. "It is my belief," he wrote in 1908, "that the time will come when not only will eugenics form an integral part of the teaching and research work of the great universities, but also will come to be regarded as a legitimate field for the Federal Government."[11] Between 1908 and 1913, he wrote seventeen articles pertaining to human heredity. After witnessing the events of the early 1920's, he came to view propaganda on eugenics differently. He complained of "its indifference to the truth"[12] and of "the feverish and frequently successful efforts of brash eugenists to influence legislation."[13] His journals reflected his new attitude. The *Quarterly Review* had an advisory board comprised of experts from fourteen fields, including "genetics," "zoology," "anthropology," and "cytology," but not "eugenics" or "human genetics." Neither journal included any material on eugenics. Through 1940, the *Quarterly Review* had published only four studies of human genetics. *Human Biology* remained sympathetic to research in human genetics—it presented work in the field often—but it primarily published statistical treatments of the subject, and the majority of the papers came from Pearl himself or from associates at the Institute for Biological Research at Johns Hopkins, which he directed. He correctly recognized that the style and use of research in human genetics of some of the more ardent devotees of the eugenics movement "is certain to have only its just effect upon the progress of human biology."[14]

While the journals were growing unhappy with human genetics, many investigators individually protested the manner in which studies in the field were frequently performed. Some of the most significant criticisms came from the pen of Harvard's William Castle. Though a mammalian geneticist, he did not contribute to the original literature of human inheritance; nevertheless he had followed developments in human genetics with great interest and for years had participated in the eugenics movement. The movement's racism in the 1920's disillusioned him with human genetics, however. He spoke out against the popularly held notion that racial crossing in man tends to produce physical deterioration, a biological argument widely used to discourage miscegenation. He wrote: "So far as a biologist can see, human race problems are not biological problems any more than rabbit crosses are social problems. The rabbit breeder does not

11. Raymond Pearl, "Breeding Better Men," *World's Work*, 15(1908):9824.
12. Raymond Pearl, "The Biology of Superiority," *The American Mercury*, 12(1927):260.
13. *Ibid.*, p. 261.
14. *Ibid.*, p. 260.

cross his selected races of rabbits unless he desires to improve upon what he has. The sociologist who is satisfied with human society as now constructed may reasonably decry race crossing. But let him do so on social grounds only. He will wait in vain, if he waits to see mixed races vanish from any biological unfitness."[15] He also harshly criticized a study of race crossing in Jamaica conducted by Davenport and Morris Steggerda, an unimaginative zoology Ph.D. After providing several examples of how the authors drew conclusions unjustified from their data, he ended:

> We like to think of the Negro as inferior. We like to think of Negro-white crosses as a degradation of the white race. We look for evidence in support of the idea and try to persuade ourselves that we have found it even when the resemblance is slight. The honestly made records of Davenport and Steggerda tell a very different story about hybrid Jamaicans from that which Davenport and Jennings tell about them in broad sweeping statements. The former will never reach the ears of eugenics propagandists and Congressional committees; the latter will be with us as the bogey man of pure-race enthusiasts for the next hundred years.[16]

It should be remembered that Davenport was Castle's close friend and former teacher as well as the man to whom he had dedicated his textbook, *Genetics and Eugenics.*

Another significant indictment of human genetics came in 1936 from a special committee of the American Neurological Association which had been instructed to investigate eugenic sterilization in the United States. Ironically, the committee's work was subsidized by a grant from the Carnegie Foundation, the same organization which had supported Davenport throughout his career at Cold Spring Harbor. After reviewing much of the literature of human genetics, particularly that pertaining to the inheritance of mental traits and psychiatric conditions, the report concluded: "It appears that not much scientifically valid work has been done on the subject of the inheritance of the diseases and conditions which have been considered. This might have been anticipated for neither psychiatry nor human genetics approach at present the status of exact sciences. It appears that most of the legislation which has been enacted so far is based more upon a desire to elevate the human race than upon proven facts."[17] The

15. William E. Castle, "Biological and Social Consequences of Race-Crossing," *Journal of Heredity,* 15(1924):368–69. This paper was reprinted in substance in the *American Journal of Physical Anthropology,* 9(1926):145, at the suggestion of Aleš Hrdlička.

16. William E. Castle, "Race Mixture and Physical Disharmonies," *Science,* 71(1930):605–6.

17. Abraham Myerson *et al.* (The Committee of the American Neurological Association for the Investigation of Eugenical Sterilization), *Eugenical Sterilization: A Reorientation of the Problem* (New York: Macmillan Co., 1936), p. 177.

committee felt that "investigation of the problem of inheritance, especially of the psychiatric conditions, has been haphazard and often inexact";[18] it suggested that "it well may be that no complete scientific approach is possible in the present state of our knowledge or rather of our ignorance."[19] It singled out work done by Davenport and members of the American eugenics school as invalid and of historical value only.[20] The report also pointed out that disillusionment with eugenicists' views on heredity had become widespread. "The leading geneticists," it wrote, "at least of America and England, have been very cautious in their pronunciamentos concerning eugenics, and it is apparent from their writings that they look with disfavor upon the sweeping statements made popularly and, to some extent, in the scientific literature concerning eugenic measures."[21]

English workers in the 1930's protested the political and social entanglements of human genetics even more vigorously than did the Americans. In that decade human genetics had become primarily an English enterprise, and investigators in that country clearly perceived that the field's political entanglements were discrediting it. J. B. S. Haldane wrote in *Heredity and Politics* (1938):

> It may well be that an increase in our knowledge will fully justify the application to man of certain measures which have led to improvements in the quality of our domestic animals. As one who is endeavoring to increase this knowledge, I can even say that I hope it will do so. But I believe that the facts concerning human heredity are far less simple than many people think them to be. And I hold that a premature application of our rather scanty knowledge will yield little result, and will merely serve to discredit the branch of science in which I am working.[22]

Lionel Penrose agreed with Haldane. Eugenics connoted something unscientific to him, and he had always distrusted its association with human genetics. At a time when money to support work in human genetics was extremely scarce, he declined a research grant because it had been offered by the Eugenics Education Society. He thought it important to keep tabs on the Society but did not wish to become a member, so he had his wife join instead.[23] His own involvement in human genetics arose through his

18. *Ibid.*, p. 181.
19. *Ibid.*, p. 181.
20. *Ibid.*, p. 88. Regarding much of the work done by Davenport and his associates, the committee complained: "The formulation has finally been Mendelian and the point of view ostensibly scientific" (p. 118).
21. *Ibid.*, p. 70.
22. J. B. S. Haldane, *Heredity and Politics* (New York: W. W. Norton and Co., 1938), pp. 8-9.
23. Conversations with Lionel Penrose, January 25 and 26, 1971.

interest in the causes of mental retardation,[24] and he recognized that the studies of the problem conducted by eugenicists were inhibiting progress in the field. "I consider the study of mental deficiency to be a branch of human biology," he wrote. "It provides a fruitful field for research when approached from this angle. In the past, however, research has been impeded by the widespread acceptance of ideas which are not in keeping with recent biological discoveries."[25]

The most outspoken on this matter was the English biologist Lancelot Hogben. When he entered the field of human genetics in 1930, he was dismayed to find that so many writers had forgotten that families transmit social and cultural as well as genetic heritages. He decided that human genetics as it then existed needed a thorough cleaning and that this could be accomplished only by placing the subject which heretofore had been dominated by political prejudice and racial folklore on a sound mathematical footing.[26] He said: "There has been so much undisciplined speculation concerning the social application of genetic principles that a writer who is concerned with the advancement of the science of human genetics may well hesitate to embark at this stage upon a discussion of the social applications of such knowledge as we now possess."[27] Human genetics, he wrote, will "gain prestige" only "when it ceases to be an apology for snobbery, selfishness, and class arrogance."[28] "The domain in which it is at present possible to foresee legitimate and fruitful applications of genetic science is that of preventive medicine. The pre-eminent need of the moment is research rather than propaganda. Whatever views one may entertain concerning the urgency of social policies based on genetic assumptions, the urgency of promptitude in developing the machinery of research in medical genetics should not be overlooked by any who have the advancement of pure science at heart."[29]

In criticizing work in human genetics, the English sometimes went a step further than the American geneticists. Though many English investigators were greatly dissatisfied with the field, some of them also attempted to offer it models of higher standards. One of the first to do so was Penrose, who in 1932 performed a widely quoted investigation of Mon-

24. Lionel S. Penrose to author, October 13, 1970.
25. Lionel Penrose, *Mental Defect* (New York: Farrar and Rinehart, 1934), p. vii.
26. Conversation with Lancelot Hogben, February 1, 1971.
27. Lancelot Hogben, *Genetic Principles in Medicine and Social Science* (New York: Alfred A. Knopf, 1932), p. 200.
28. Lancelot Hogben, *Science for the Citizen* (New York: Alfred A. Knopf, 1938), p. 1061. See also Lancelot Hogben, *Nature and Nurture*, rev. ed. (New York: W. W. Norton and Co., 1939), p. 33.
29. Hogben, *Genetic Principles*, p. 214.

golian idiocy as a case study of how the interrelated factors of heredity and environment should be analyzed in studies of human genetics. It is worth quoting in detail from the introduction to his paper:

> Most studies of human genetics which have hitherto been made have not taken into consideration the full significance of the environmental influences which may modify the data from which numerical conclusions have been drawn. Some early geneticists, like Bateson, confined their attention to what appeared to be simple physical characters, like brachydactyly and eye colour. In later studies, however, now that the field of such simple phenomena is becoming exhausted, attacks have been made by the same methods on problems of an entirely different nature. Studies in the inheritance of acquired diseases, like tuberculosis, would be cases in point. And, while few people would be foolish enough to suppose, for example, that a study of affected and normal members of tuberculous families would give numerical results which could be utilised as those of brachydactyly, it is surprising how many observers have treated the more subtle phenomenon of mental disease in ways which are open to severest criticism. It is, moreover, probable that a very large class of human characteristics of a directly physical nature are determined to a considerable extent by environmental influences, although they may also give evidence of being phenomena suitable for genetic investigation. . . . But, although such problems are well understood in experimental genetics, little serious attempt has so far been made to tackle them as far as human beings are concerned.
>
> The present paper sets out to describe some methods which may be of use in making such an attempt, and the example of 'mongolian' imbecility is taken to show how the methods can be applied in practice.[30]

A similar work was Hogben's 1932 book, *Genetic Principles in Medicine and Social Science*, in which he denounced much of the work being done in human genetics and pleaded for caution in the application of genetic principles to human affairs. In the book he expressed great dissatisfaction with the methods and approaches commonly employed in the field:

> Writers on human genetics have hitherto devoted very little attention to the requirements of a rigorous treatment of genetically determined conditions. They have been content to compile data from studies in fraternal and filial correlation or from family pedigrees. The technique of correlation, properly controlled, and appropriately applied to properly authenticated data, is a useful instrument for certain kinds of investigation, especially the study of twin resemblance. . . . The fact that it is almost universally overlooked by biological writers is not calculated to increase

---

30. Lionel S. Penrose, "On the Interaction of Heredity and Environment in the Study of Human Genetics' (with Special Reference to Mongolian Imbecility)," *Journal of Genetics*, 25(1932):407–8.

the confidence with which others envisage the possibility of making human genetics a progressive and precise body of human knowledge. If this book calls forth the strictures of those biologists who are disposed to exaggerate the importance of hereditary differences, the author is confident that he will encourage others who have been alienated by this unfortunate bias to adopt a more sympathetic attitude to the study of hereditary transmission in human beings.[31]

He was especially critical of those human geneticists who permitted the discipline to be misused for political purposes:

At a time when we hear so much of the superiority of the Nordic race, it may be well to bear in mind the views of those who were preparing the ground for the cultural development of Northern Europe when our own forbears were little better than barbarians. . . .

Fortunately the study of human genetics is becoming sufficiently complex to encourage the hope that it will soon be removed from the atmosphere of the drawing-room to that of the laboratory. If this book assists in accomplishing the divorce of a genuinely scientific study of genetic influences in human society from amateur political speculation, it will have achieved as much as its author can hope.[32]

Though he felt that medical uses could be found for human genetics, he preferred the term "genetic therapy" to "eugenics" for this province of applied human genetics, since:

The term "eugenics" has become identified with ancestor worship, antisemitism, colour prejudice, antifeminism, snobbery, and obstruction to educational progress. Whatever may be said for such views, they are not the inevitable consequence of biological study, and whatever residuum of salutary maxims is implied in the strictly etymological significance of the term, eugenics has long since acquired associations which are repugnant to many thoughtful persons, whether biologically trained or not.[33]

Hogben developed these themes again the following year in *Nature and Nurture*.

A futher indication of how the excesses of eugenicists impeded progress in human genetics could be seen during the "takeoff" of human genetics at the end of World War II. At that time several journals in the fields of eugenics and human genetics began or resumed publication, and in their editorial prefaces many of these pointed to the uncritical work of the pre-Depression years as the epitome of research that must be *avoided* if

31. Hogben, *Genetic Principles*, pp. 9–10.
32. *Ibid.*, pp. 213–14.
33. *Ibid.*, p. 209.

human genetics were to become a legitimate science. In the introductory issue of *The American Journal of Human Genetics*, H. J. Muller, the first president of the American Society of Human Genetics, criticized much of the early work and blamed it for markedly retarding interest in the field. After examining at length the misconceptions and errors made by the early workers, he concluded:

> All this patent forcing of the data, and, still more so, of the interpretations, led many critically minded persons to look askance at both the specific and general claims made. Even more so did the fact that these precarious conclusions were often used in support of sweeping recommendations for eugenic measures, and that many of the studies were little more than accessories, made to put forward the preconceived eugenic notions of the writers.
>
> Quite obviously the cart had been put before the horse, to the detriment of both. It would be helpful, for those now intending to work in this field, to examine some of these early reports critically, as object lessons of what procedures to avoid.[34]

Finally, after World War II, warnings against the errors made by eugenicists began to appear in many textbooks of genetics and human genetics. Laurence H. Snyder told readers of his *Human Genetics* (fourth edition, 1951) of the early eugenicists' mistakes and prejudices:

> Unfortunately, too, it was almost inevitable that a movement whose program predicated the evaluation of innate superiority and inferiority should attract many persons with strong prejudices regarding the special status of their own race, nation, or social group. It is undeniable that the constructive aims of eugenics have drawn into the movement many who have been motivated by exclusively altruistic considerations; but it is equally undeniable that the eugenics movement has been severely handicapped throughout its history by adherents who have been more conspicuous for enthusiasm than for critical acumen. . . .
>
> The foregoing discussion indicates that we should hesitate at accepting without careful analysis the claims and recommendations that are presented in a large portion of the eugenics literature. It also suggests why professionally trained geneticists, on the whole, have given relatively little support to eugenic theories and programs. A number of prominent geneticists in fact, including T. H. Morgan, H. S. Jennings, T. Dobzhansky, L. C. Dunn, Lancelot Hogben, J. B. S. Haldane, and H. J. Muller, have been explicitly critical, with varying degrees of vigor, of substantial portions of orthodox eugenic doctrine.[35]

34. H. J. Muller, "Progress and Prospects in Human Genetics," *The American Journal of Human Genetics*, 1(1949):6–7.

35. Laurence H. Snyder, *The Principles of Heredity*, 4th ed. (Boston: D. C. Health Co., 1951), pp. 436–37.

In *Human Heredity* (1954), after recounting the "lurid and disquieting history" of the eugenics movement, James V. Neel and William J. Schull stressed: "It is imperative that in this renewal of interest [in the modern eugenics movement] the lessons of the past be not forgotten. Every sincere believer in the development of eugenics would do well to refer from time to time to such biased presentations of the problem as Grant's *Passing of the Great Race*, as a reminder of the extremes to which so-called 'eugenicists' of other days have gone and the pitfalls to be avoided."[36] The anthropologist Ashley Montagu wrote in *Human Heredity* (1959), a popular treatise:

> There are many people, some honestly well-meaning and others dubiously so, who maintain that the restriction of immigration to "desirable types" and the "sterilization of the unfit" would greatly benefit our society. Unfortunately the voices of such individuals have sometimes made themselves so effectively heard that they have influenced national and state policies. It is perhaps not as well known as it should be that the United States Immigration Act of 1924 was based on the ill-considered, prejudiced, and unscientific judgments of the late Mr. Harry Laughlin, a worker in The Eugenics Records Office at Cold Spring Harbor, New York, supported behind the scenes by Madison Grant, the author of the notorious *The Passing of the Great Race*, and Charles Benedict Davenport, the Director of the Office, to whose remarkable judgment on matters racial in his *Race Crossing in Jamaica* reference has already been made.[37]

He also complained of Laughlin's influence in passing sterilization bills.[38]

Examples such as these indicate dramatically how human genetics' entanglement with eugenics contributed to the field's slow progress between 1920 and 1940. Human genetics had become burdened with the stigma of eugenics. Many journals and organizations concerned with human genetics either renounced their association with eugenics or disappeared. Warnings against eugenics and criticisms of work in human genetics appeared in the technical literature of human genetics, occasionally in more popular publications, and eventually in textbooks on the subject. There were men in the late 1920's and 1930's who turned away from the field because they had grown unhappy with its political involvements. Moreover, even some investigators who did contribute to the field did little to encourage others to

36. James V. Neel and William J. Schull, *Human Heredity* (Chicago: The University of Chicago Press, 1954), p. 337.

37. Ashley Montagu, *Human Heredity* (Cleveland: World Publishing Co., 1959), p. 288. See also pp. 25–26.

38. *Ibid.*, pp. 288–89.

enter it. Though Muller, for instance, had a life-long interest in guiding man's genetic future and made important original contributions himself to the subject,[39] in the laboratory he studied Drosophila exclusively and did not encourage his graduate students to enter human genetics. Those of his students who later did do work in the field, such as Oliver, generally became interested in doing so through other influences after they had left Muller's laboratory.[40]

It is difficult to compare the extent to which political misuse hindered human genetics with the degree in which technical problems impeded it. One may wonder what contributions to the subject Herbert Jennings, a protozoan geneticist, might have made had he not been forced to join his colleagues in voicing unhappiness with the field. It is important to keep in mind, however, that the consequences of the field's political entanglements cannot be measured simply in terms of well-known geneticists who stopped contributing new material to human genetics. Rather, it must be recognized that geneticists' biting criticisms of the field constituted a negative judgment from the elite of the science regarding the respectability of human genetics as an area of research. In choosing a specialty, young investigators quite naturally solicit the advice of senior men on what fields hold the most promise for discovery and personal fulfillment. How many young men might otherwise have been tempted to enter human genetics in the 1930's had not so many "elders" of the day failed to endorse the field as a deserving scientific enterprise!

Thus, the intemperance of many eugenicists in their quest to enact legislation had a dual effect on genetics: it prompted the development of a sense of social responsibility among many geneticists, and it retarded progress in the study of human heredity. Early workers in human genetics did not possess a monopoly on bias; prejudice could be found even among their most astute critics. As Hogben admitted: "A scientific worker is also a human being, and shares many of the prejudices and limitations of other human beings. If he can get outside some of them when he is inside the

39. Muller's most important original contribution to human genetics was an article entitled "Mental Traits and Heredity" which appeared in the *Journal of Heredity* in 1925. In this paper he attempted to show the extent to which mental traits are independent of heredity, using a case of identical twins reared apart.

40. Clarence P. Oliver to author, August 4, 1970.

While the great majority of Muller's students became Drosophila experimentalists like their mentor, they were keenly aware of the issues raised by the social applications of heredity and frequently discussed these questions among themselves. (Conversation with James F. Crow, September 22, 1970. Crow was a student of Wilson J. Stone, who obtained his degree under Muller.)

laboratory, he is still entitled to likes and dislikes."[41] Unfortunately, however, many early workers in human genetics committed the cardinal error of not sufficiently casting their presuppositions aside when entering the laboratory. An investigator's scientific judgment will not necessarily be biased by a desire to see his findings applied to human affairs, but that is what happened to too many early eugenic enthusiasts pursuing human genetics. The result was a period of great suspicion and distrust of the motives of almost everyone involved with the field.

2. English vs. American Geneticists

In the 1930's a cloud of suspicion hovered over the field of human genetics; groups of geneticists reacted to that situation in varying ways. One group of geneticists remained as interested in human genetics and eugenics as ever. So far as these men could see, there was no reason to regard the field of human genetics with displeasure. This group was small in size, and its best-known members were Davenport, Laughlin, Gates, and Popenoe. (Popenoe did not have a graduate degree in biology, but he spoke to the public as a biologist and from 1913 to 1917 edited the *Journal of Heredity*.) A second group regarded the field of human genetics with such great suspicion that it turned away from the discipline. Among its members were individuals who themselves had once contributed to human genetics or the eugenics movement. Almost all the first-generation American geneticists, including men like Morgan, Jennings, Pearl, Castle, and East, belonged to this group. A third group shared the majority's dissatisfaction with what had happened in human genetics but nonetheless retained interest and hope in it. With fresh enthusiasm they made new contributions to the field and offered their work as models of how studies in human inheritance should be conducted. This group consisted mainly of a small number of young English investigators, the most notable of whom were Hogben, Haldane, Penrose, R. A. Fisher, and Fraser Roberts. The Americans H. J. Muller and Laurence H. Snyder also belonged here. I shall now seek to identify what distinguished these three groups and what accounted for their varied attitudes toward human genetics.

The most obvious difference was between members of the first group and those of the second and third. Persons in the first group, unlike the rest, were biased and closed-minded individuals whose social views greatly influenced their interpretation of scientific evidence. History and the so-

41. Lancelot Hogben, *Author in Transit* (New York: W. W. Norton and Co., 1940), p. 14.

cial context, of course, help determine every scientist's choice of problems. It also is possible for an investigator to do objective science and still be interested in its social consequences. Individuals in this first group, however, possessed social biases strong enough to produce gross aberrations in their critical judgment as measured by the standards of their peers. Even in the 1940's they espoused an outmoded view of the process of inheritance which said simply that heredity is more important than environment and that almost all traits obey Mendel's laws. Most of these individuals were bigots; a few even applauded Hitler. They used their scientific theories to support their social views, which were those commonly held by eugenicists. Almost all their contemporaries distrusted their motives and considered their research too biased to be of value.[42]

Laughlin typified this group. Despite an Sc.D. from Princeton in 1917, he never achieved a feeling for the methods and values of science. His work was so unsound, his conclusions so dominated by his prejudices that he became a laughingstock to many of his fellow biologists. As Davenport's assistant at Cold Spring Harbor, he channeled most of his energy not into scientific pursuits but into political activism; first the state sterilization laws, then the Immigration Restriction Act. He seemed to lack the discipline and objectivity of a scientist, and his attempts at genetics showed little common sense or critical judgment. He was a humorless individual, intolerant of criticism, extremely unapproachable and reserved, and little liked by others. He became obsessed with the idea of passing laws and approached the eugenics crusade passionately.[43]

Davenport stood apart from others in this group, for he possessed a genuinely scientific temperament. Though he occasionally lectured or signed petitions in behalf of eugenic legislation, he was primarily a scientist who had little use for eugenic propaganda. As he told Mrs. E. M. East, he

42. Note that the majority or accepted view is not necessarily the correct or unbiased one. In his views on race Franz Boas for many years stood virtually alone and a generation ahead of other American anthropologists of the day.

43. It would seem that hard-line eugenicists like Laughlin genuinely believed they were in possession of Absolute Truth. Historically, such persons have tended to be end-oriented rather than means-oriented, hence fundamentally undemocratic if not overtly anti-democratic in their approach. Moses and Jesus hardly subjected their rules to the popular approbation of the masses. Absolute Truth can tolerate no dissent. Dissent, under such circumstances, constitutes heresy. Anti-democratic attitudes were held by many of the hard-line eugenicists. See, for example, Madison Grant, "Discussion of Article on Democracy and Heredity," *Journal of Heredity*, 10(1919):164; and Prescott F. Hall, "Aristocracy and Politics," *Journal of Heredity*, 10(1919):166. The views presented in these two articles may be compared with the democratic attitudes expressed by Edwin G. Conklin, a much less zealous eugenicist, in "Heredity and Democracy," *Journal of Heredity*, 10(1919):161.

found it desirable "to decline to associate myself with any sort of propaganda, even propaganda on eugenics."[44] He said to her: "You are beginning on the wrong end in working for broader and saner laws and secondly, upon research. . . . I am inclined to think that we should first make an investigation to see if there are any definite historical data and then make use of such data in drawing a conclusion to whether legislation be desirable or not."[45] Unlike others in this group, he was not a racist; he customarily spoke of minorities in an objective and circumspect manner. He was an exceptionally kind individual who helped many young investigators get their starts in biology. When Curt Stern decided not to return to Germany in 1933, Davenport provided him a temporary position and repeatedly journeyed to the railroad station himself to provide transportation for the young Stern without even considering to send a subordinate.[46] He enjoyed amicable relations with most of his colleagues, and even so careful a worker as T. H. Morgan held him in great respect.

Though some of Davenport's later work might have been laughed at, Davenport the man was not. Early in his career he had earned plaudits for his contributions to ecology and statistics as well as for his better efforts in human genetics. All his work, however, suffered from what one colleague has called his "pioneering temperament."[47] He was supremely skilled at recognizing the broad importance of a field but not at following through in the details of research. He was imbued with too little patience and persistence to stick to a topic and work out the details to others' satisfaction; he tended to jump to conclusions on the basis of inadequate evidence and pass on to whatever subject next captured his attention. This "hit and run" approach characterized some of his work with animals, such as his poultry experiments, as well as his work with human problems. His contemporaries consequently regarded him as a "pioneer type"; they respected him more for public relations and for getting things going in a field than for his personal contributions to the literature. Davenport still remains an enigma, however, because a "pioneering temperament" does not completely explain why he failed to acknowledge the more complex picture of inheritance portrayed by later work of clarification and expansion in genetics. He was considered a reasonable man; he was not overly sensitive to criticism; yet throughout his career he remained convinced of

44. C. B. Davenport to Mrs. E. M. East, November 10, 1916, *CBD*.
45. *Ibid.*
46. Conversation with Curt Stern, September 29, 1970.
47. Conversation with Sewall Wright, September 24, 1970.

the basic correctness of his views regarding human inheritance. Whatever his reasons were, he maintained the appearance of a man of science which others in this group failed to do.

Members of the latter two groups differed greatly from those of the first. They too, of course, were not unbiased when discussing the social applications of genetics, a fact which did not escape their notice. Hogben pointed out: "Biologists cannot be expected to be free from ethical preferences. They are entitled to the same allowance of prejudices as the private citizen."[48] Some of them also disliked particular minorities. East used to complain bitterly to his laboratory workers of the "corrupt" Irish who dominated Boston politics.[49] Whatever their presuppositions, nevertheless, they managed to keep their social and scientific views reasonably apart. Among their ranks were men of the political left and right and persons of widely varying views toward the questions raised by eugenicists. None of them permitted their feelings on social matters to compromise their scientific judgment to such a degree that they failed to meet the standard of objectivity accepted by their peers. They remained free enough of their personal biases so that they could properly and critically interpret scientific evidence, including that which related to man. They retained the ability to change their minds when new evidence appeared.

Castle exemplified these qualities. Underneath a certain formality to his manner was a kindly, open, sympathetic nature. A pugnacious investigator, one of the important defenders of Mendelism during its controversy with biometry, he had a career marked by continual dispute, particularly with the Morgan school over some of the subsidiary hypotheses of the chromosome theory of heredity. In these controversies Castle was often wrong, but he quickly and graciously admitted his mistakes as soon as he recognized them. One time he was led by his own experiments to see the error in a certain view of selection and gene variability which he had vigorously defended for nearly twenty years. L. C. Dunn, who was a student of Castle's, recalls the occasion:

Characteristically he made the correction in a seminar attended by his students and colleagues, some of whom had previously voiced their disagreement with his earlier interpretation. He introduced his remarks by saying that when he had told his wife that morning that he was to "correct" his long held views about selection, she had commented that he had

48. Hogben, *Genetic Principles*, p. 36.
49. Conversation with R. A. Brink, September 22, 1970. Brink was a graduate student under East.

spent a good deal of time recently in unsaying what he had said in previous years. "I agree," said Castle, "and consider that it represents progress."[50]

As seen earlier, this erstwhile eugenic enthusiast showed the same ability to modify his views on matters relating to eugenics and human inheritance.

Intellectual, historical, and sociological reasons accounted for the differences between the second and third groups. The most visible distinction between them was the intellectual one: the two groups attacked genetic problems in characteristically different manners. The second group, which in the 1930's became disillusioned with human genetics, consisted primarily of experimental geneticists, whereas the third group, which continued to pursue the field, was comprised largely of statistical geneticists. Experimentalists had always tended to shy away from human genetics because of the obvious difficulties in dealing with a species which breeds slowly, produces few offspring, and mates for its own rather than for the investigator's satisfaction. Because of these problems, plus the difficulty in distinguishing a homozygous from a heterozygous parent, problems which might be trivial in experimental genetics—such as linkage analysis and gene mapping—became formidable in human genetics. Attempts to apply the experimental method to man were frustrating and usually unsuccessful, and accordingly most experimental geneticists channeled their efforts into other areas—particularly Drosophila genetics, whose enormous advance by the 1920's had smothered everything else.

Despite these problems, early studies in human genetics successfully discovered certain pathological traits showing striking phenotypic discontinuities which behave as Mendelian characteristics. By the 1920's and 1930's the supply of such characteristics had been greatly exhausted, however, and more sophisticated methods were needed to handle traits which showed no such conspicuous discontinuities or which followed more complex patterns of hereditary transmission. At this point future progress in human genetics depended upon the development of sophisticated statistical techniques to deal with these matters. Fortunately for the science, the period between 1917 and 1932 witnessed the rise of statistical and population genetics, much of which was developed through the use of human populations as examples.[51] Population genetics involved the application of rigorous mathematical and analytical methods to working out the consequences of Mendelian heredity in populations of plants, animals, and men.

50. L. C. Dunn, "William Ernest Castle," *National Academy of Sciences of the United States, Biographical Memoirs*, 38(1965):44.

51. For an account of the development of population genetics see L. C. Dunn, *A Short History of Genetics* (New York: McGraw-Hill 1965), chapters 12 and 20.

With these methods information could be obtained concerning such phenomena as evolutionary mechanisms, the frequency and behavior of genes in populations, and the inheritance of "biometrical" or "quantitative" traits. The groundwork of population genetics had been established in 1908 by Hardy and Weinberg, but for nearly a decade no one appreciated the significance of their work. (Indeed, not until 1943, when the Hardy-Weinberg law received its present name, did Weinberg's contribution gain general recognition.[52]) Until 1917 the leading statistician was Karl Pearson, but his methods were simple and soon to be supplemented, and his work suffered greatly by his insistence that Mendelism is incorrect. In 1917 Sewall Wright rediscovered Hardy's equilibrium principle, and during the next fifteen years he, along with Haldane and R. A. Fisher, extended the equation to develop the theoretical basis of modern population genetics. Through the 1930's most work in the area was theoretical, not yet tested experimentally with plant or animal populations. The one major exception was studies on the human blood groups by Levine, Wiener, Hirszfeld, Snyder, Bernstein, Race, and others. The ABO blood types provided human genetics a set of "test characters" for analysis and demonstrated the importance to the science of gene-frequency analyses in particular and statistical methods in general. Snyder has suggested that "the blood groups have been to human genetics what Drosophila has been to classical genetics."[53]

Most members of the third group were pioneers in applying the new statistical methods to human genetics, and those of them who were not, such as Muller, were at least familiar and comfortable with basic statistical techniques. They recognized that little progress in the future would be made solely by compiling pedigrees of rare traits, and they urged that human genetics be made quantitative. When Penrose entered human genetics in the early 1930's, the atmosphere was completely ignorant and amateurish. He was especially vexed by the customary attempts to apply strict Mendelian methods to human material. He recognized from the start that it is self-defeating to try to do so unless one is working with traits that Mendelize. His attention turned to statistical analyses of human inheritance, an approach he felt had already proceeded far enough to lay the foundation of a legitimate science of human genetics applicable to medical problems.[54] Fraser Roberts had begun his career as a biologist and animal

52. The Hardy-Weinberg law was named by Curt Stern in 1943. See Stern, "The Hardy-Weinberg Law," *Science*, 97(1943):137.
53. Laurence H. Snyder, "Old and New Pathways in Human Genetics," in L. C. Dunn, ed., *Genetics in the 20th Century* (New York: Macmillan Co., 1951), p. 371.
54. Conversation with Lionel Penrose, January 25, 1971.

geneticist for the Wool Industries Research Association, and from the start he too had been statistically minded and interested in analyses of measurement. Fisher, his friend and benefactor, and F. A. E. Crew, his first chief, increased his appetite for statistics even further and stimulated his interest in human genetics. After obtaining an M.D. degree for research purposes, he began to perform statistical investigations of human heredity.[55] Crew, who has written several books on human genetics, was not statistically equipped himself; nevertheless he believed that such an approach to human genetics was necessary, and he frequently collaborated with expert statisticians. At different times Roberts and Hogben both worked with him.[56]

Some of these men publicly exhorted others to join them in developing statistical methods for human genetics. Haldane wrote in his *New Paths in Genetics* (1942), "I have tried to show how, in the study of human genetics, statistical methods replace the various technical devices, such as milk bottles and etherizers, which are familiar to the *Drosophila* worker. . . . they are essential adjuncts to any study of human genetics which goes beyond the mere accumulation of pedigrees."[57] Hogben had entered human genetics with the hope of making it respectable, and he thought that the only way to accomplish this was to make it quantitative.[58] He pointed out that "little progress will be made in genetical analysis of pathological traits by compilation of recorded data."[59] He felt: "To-day [1932] the prospects for advancing Human Genetics as an exact science are much brighter than they appeared to be twenty years ago. New methods of mathematical analysis for testing the applicability of experimentally established hypotheses to human data have been elaborated. On the basis of such work as Bernstein's analysis of the blood groups it is now legitimate to entertain the possibility that the human chromosome can be mapped."[60] Snyder wrote in 1933:

No longer does the familiar 3:1 ratio cover the major portion of the field of heredity. As a matter of fact, ratios of the sort found in the F_2 generations of animals and plants are not observable as such in man. No single human family is large enough, as a rule, to provide a valid ratio in any generation. And when groups of families are lumped together for analysis, aberrant ratios are obtained because it is usually impossible to

55. Conversation with Fraser Roberts, January 27, 1971.
56. Conversation with F. A. E. Crew, February 4, 1971.
57. J. B. S. Haldane, *New Paths in Genetics* (New York: Harper and Brothers, 1942), p. 194.
58. Conversation with Lancelot Hogben, February 1, 1971.
59. Lancelot Hogben, "The Genetic Analysis of Familial Traits. I. Single Gene Substitutions," *Journal of Genetics*, 25(1931):112.
60. Hogben, *Genetic Principles*, p. 214.

separate homozygous parents from heterozygous parents. This leads to a radically diffirent type of analysis of human pedigrees, the study of the frequencies of the factors concerned. This method of analysis promises far-reaching benefits to medicine in the future.[61]

These men spoke as much as prophets and reformers as they did as investigators; the power of their statistical techniques had imbued them with new confidence and optimism regarding the future progress of human genetics.

It is important to appreciate how greatly these two approaches, the statistical and the experimental, varied. The pencil and paper world of the theoretical, statistical geneticist was unfamiliar and uncomfortable to the Drosophila experimentalist accustomed to milk bottles and etherizers. Both approaches had intellectual rigor, but of their own sorts. Such a superb experimentalist as Castle, for instance, who was highly skilled at reducing complex hypotheses to simple testable experiments, regarded abstractions with suspicion and frequently made mistakes with problems requiring the use of mathematics or statistics.[62] Though investigators in the 1920's and 1930's tended to be less specialized than workers today, so radically did these two approaches differ that only a few exceptional individuals could pursue them both successfully.

This discussion also suggests why human genetics in the 1930's was essentially a British property: the leading statisticians—Haldane, Hogben, Fisher, Penrose, Yule, Pearson—all were on the eastern side of the Atlantic. Davenport and Pearl used statistics, but their methods were of the earlier Karl Pearson era. They never became adept at the more powerful procedures developed later, and they did not make any significant contributions to human genetics methodology. Snyder did admirable work, but he was not a Fisher or Haldane. The one American at this time of comparable statistical inventiveness to the British was Sewall Wright, who was more interested in guinea pigs and evolution than in man.[63] In other words, in the 1930's the methods capable of making human genetics scientifically

---

61. Laurence H. Snyder, "Genetics and Medicine," *The Ohio State Medical Journal*, 29(1933):706.

62. Dunn, "William Ernest Castle," p. 56; Sewall Wright, "William Ernest Castle, 1867–1962," *Genetics*, 48(1963):4.

63. Wright has written only one paper on human genetics, but an aversion of his to the field should not be inferred. When he came to the University of Chicago in 1925, his small department already had one member working in human genetics. Though no one hinted or suggested the idea to him, he felt that the interests of the department could best be served if he performed his population studies with some organism other than man. Ironically, when he arrived at Chicago he considered himself a physiological geneticist first and a population geneticist only second. After all, he had trained under William Castle. So many people wrote to him with population

respectable had been mastered and employed mainly by the British. Haldane was accustomed to remarking that aside from himself there were only half a dozen people in the world who knew anything about human genetics,[64] and with the exception of Gunnar Dahlberg they were all English.

Another reason for the contrasting attitudes of the second and third groups toward human genetics was that the historical situation of the English eugenics movement differed from that of the American movement.[65] For several reasons eugenics hindered human genetics less in England than in the United States. First, the Eugenics Education Society, the principal English eugenics organization, was much less overtly racist than counterpart organizations in America. It was also less vocally and articulately pro-Nazi. This was understandable since England lacked the immigrant and Negro populations which prompted such a marked racial consciousness among American eugenicists. The English eugenics movement was characterized instead by a temperament peculiarly fuedalistic. From its beginning the Eugenics Education Society largely consisted of a collection of social snobs very conscious of "being well born" who expressed silly views on heredity. To most observers they appeared foolish and haughty, but few onlookers thought of them as pernicious.

Moreover, the English eugenics movement, unlike the American movement, never had any significant political influence. Despite its resources and wealth (many benefactors, thinking they were helping to improve the human race, bequeathed large sums to the Eugenics Education Society), the movement was politically impotent and never came close to obtaining a sterilization law. Only a small but vocal minority among the well-to-do supported its political goals. The masses, offended by eugenicists' unconcealed snobbery, could not be persuaded to do so. Class consciousness had saturated almost all eugenic writing in England and had deprived the movement of any possible political power.[66]

---

and statistical problems, however, that he found he could not get out, and statistical work in this way became his first line of research. (Conversation with Sewall Wright, September 24, 1970.)

64. Lionel Penrose to author, October 13, 1970.

65. Impressions on the English eugenics movement were obtained in conversations with Lionel Penrose, Lancelot Hogben, Fraser Roberts, F. A. E. Crew, and Harry Harris.

66. Penrose recalls that the propagandizing of the Eugenics Education Society caused him difficulty in his medical work. In the early 1930's eugenicists traveled around England lecturing to the public that parents of children of less than normal intelligence should be sterilized. Penrose would then encounter hostility from parents of mental defectives he was treating because they had heard such a lecture and suspected that he was going to recommended that they should be sterilized! (Conversation with Lionel Penrose, January 25, 1971.)

The English eugenics movement, furthermore, never enjoyed significant scientific influence. Whereas eugenics in America had always been associated with the Mendelians, the roots of the movement in England were biometrical, and eugenics in that country had from the start come to be identified with biometry, Galton, and Pearson. Experimentalists in England immediately washed their hands of it, not because they disputed eugenics ideologically, but because of their distaste with biometry. The biometricians after a while also came to distrust the eugenicists, however, and Pearson and Galton themselves felt compelled to stress that no organic connection existed between the Galton Laboratory and the Eugenics Education Society.[67] Thus, eugenics in England quite early lost favor among all the leading geneticists, the biometricians as well as the Mendelians. This circumstance had a significant consequence for the development of human genetics in that country. In England there had been a long, established interest in the field among both Mendelians and biometricians, neither of whom were closely associated with the eugenics movement after the falling out between the Galton Laboratory and the Eugenics Society. The alliance between eugenics and human genetics in that country became very tenuous; human genetics in England no longer so clearly constituted the province of "pure eugenics" as it had been before the two organizations parted ways. Though many English workers in the area continued for decades afterwards to be influenced by eugenic biases, and though much work in the field continued to be done by amateurs, the more astute English geneticists saw a bit earlier than the Americans that the fate of human genetics did not have to be wrapped up with that of eugenics.

The final distinction between the second and third groups was sociological. As seen earlier, members of the second group, first-generation American geneticists born primarily in the 1860's and 1870's, believed strongly in the concept of "biological sociology"—the idea of using science as method and of looking to biology for guidance in solving social problems. This was understandable for a group of men who were born and reared as Darwinism was rapidly diffusing into popular thought and who generally arose from the same middle-class strata of society that produced the majority of that generation's scientists, engineers, physicians, professors, lawyers, educators, and progressives. As proponents of biological sociology, their vision of human genetics had from the start merged with their hopes for the eugenics movement. They did not think of human

67. Karl Pearson records the events which led to the parting of the ways of the Galton Laboratory and the Eugenics Education Society in Pearson, *The Life, Letters, and Labours of Francis Galton*, vol. 3-a (London: Cambridge University Press, 1930), pp. 404–9.

genetics as a separate, objective, independent discipline existing apart from eugenics; they did not consider it a science in its own right as they did chemistry, physics, or even conventional genetics. Rather, they regarded research in human genetics as investigation in "pure eugenics," as a way to determine the guidelines for future eugenic programs. As long as their commitment to biological sociology remained, they were incapable of viewing human genetics as anything else.

After World War I, naturalism, Social Darwinism, and Herbert Spencer rapidly lost influence in America. The war did much to quench their popularity. It destroyed the faith of many individuals in the inevitability of progress, an essential component of the naturalistic world view. It also ended admiration for rugged Darwinian individualism, which many Americans felt was typified by Germany's "philosophy of force" and "nationalistic militarism." Biological sociology managed to survive this initial onslaught upon naturalism, but it did not survive the 1930's when the economic chaos of that decade made absurd the analogy between society and organism and the claim that only biological law is at work in the social fabric. The Depression also showed strict laissez-faire capitalism and individualism to be unworkable in the United States and forced many to accept the idea of governmental planning and collective security.

Though biological sociology was declining in influence after the war, it retained its importance to many first-generation geneticists. So strong was their belief in this philosophy that many of them *never* abandoned it. In *1936* Samuel Holmes had these words of praise for the ideas of Herbert Spencer:

When Herbert Spencer wrote his well-known book on *The Study of Sociology* he devoted a chapter to showing that sociology rests upon biological foundations and that preparation in biology is therefore necessary for the proper cultivation of the social sciences. The progress of biology has yielded abundant support for this conclusion and has shown that the connections between biology and sociology are more numerous and intimate than was probably appreciated even by Spencer.[68]

He continued:

We face many problems of social biology that urgently call for solution. What shall be done with the hereditarily defective classes? How shall we control immigration in the best interest of future generations? In what ways can we hope to overcome the evils of the differential birth rate? These and many other questions bring us face to face with issues upon

68. Samuel J. Holmes, *Human Genetics and its Social Import* (New York: McGraw-Hill 1936), p. v.

which we find people stoutly maintaining opposing views. We cannot answer any of these questions without some knowledge of genetics. They are social problems, but they can be solved only by a study of biological facts.[69]

Holmes was not an isolated example. During the 1920's, 1930's, and even the 1940's, similar views were expressed by many geneticists of his generation. Conklin wrote in 1921:

In considering the bearings of evolution upon government and religion, I realize that I am dealing with subjects which are generally regarded as quite outside the field of biology. However, I am convinced that nothing which concerns man is wholly foreign to the fundamental principles of life and evolution, and that the future progress of mankind depends upon a rational application of the principle of science to all human affairs.[70]

East prefaced a book in 1927 by stating his belief that principles of heredity "may be of service in analyzing some of the more important social questions."[71] He felt that "the established facts concerning variations, heredity, and development provide a new orientation in sociology."[72] Jennings introduced his wide-selling *Biological Basis of Human Nature* (1930) by proposing to answer the questions: "What has biology to say that is of interest to men, not as zoologists or botanists, but as human beings? What has biology to contribute to the understanding of our lives and of the world in which we live?"[73] Guyer wrote in 1942:

Our whole social and industrial order is ultimately, indeed, a biological problem. Unquestionably the only way toward a richer, happier life is through biologically right conduct based on trustworthy experiences arrived at by the method of science instead of through the mere wishful thinking with which we commonly beguile ourselves. Above all it is important for us to see through the eyes of science, as well as from moral precepts, the survival value of virtue. But obviously the first necessity is to learn what biological righteousness is.[74]

69. *Ibid.*, p. vi.
70. Edwin G. Conklin, *The Direction of Human Evolution*, 2nd ed. (New York: Charles Scribner's Sons, 1921), p. vii.
71. Edward M. East, *Heredity and Human Affairs* (New York: Charles Scribner's Sons, 1927), p. v.
72. *Ibid.*, p. v.
73. Herbert S. Jennings, *The Biological Basis of Human Nature* (New York: W. W. Norton and Co., 1930), p. xvii. Jennings later became more critical of the validity of biological sociology. See Jennings, "Biology and Social Reform," *Journal of Social Philosophy*, 2(1937):155.
74. Michael F. Guyer, *Speaking of Man. A Biologist Looks at Man* (New York: Harper and Brothers, 1942), p. 3.

Throughout their lives, therefore, these men endorsed the principle of biological sociology. They were deeply imbued with the intellectual bias of the upper-middle and professional classes of their generation. As they became critical of the eugenics movement in the 1920's and 1930's, they lost interest in the field of human genetics. With their faith in eugenics destroyed, most of them saw nothing else in human genetics they considered worthy of saving.[75]

The third group held strikingly different opinions of biological sociology. Members of this group came from the next generation of geneticists. Muller was born in 1890; Haldane, 1892; Hogben, 1895; Penrose, 1898; Roberts, 1899; and Snyder, 1901. Youths during World War I, young men when the Depression began, they recognized that impersonal economic forces as well as biological ones operate in society, and accordingly they rejected biological sociology as part of their own philosophies. Though they were just as disgruntled as their seniors with much of the earlier work in human genetics, their repudiation of biological sociology permitted them to envision the science as an important area of biology apart from eugenics, and they set forth to establish it as an intellectually respectable field.

Among these men Hogben most persistently voiced objections to biological sociology. His view on the matter was greatly influenced by the outpouring of what he terms "nauseating race propaganda" that he had witnessed during his stay in South Africa as a professor of zoology at the University of Capetown. He had arrived in South Africa in 1926 around the time the Afrikaners assumed power, and he was present in the country when the basic apartheid legislation was enacted. He sat in the visitors' chambers while the two houses passed the laws which deprived the natives of their political rights, including the right of assembly. He so sympathized with the natives that he publicly protested these proceedings and thereby became a marked man politically. Not wanting his children to grow up in a country which treated the black man that way, he returned to England in

75. Naturalism involved a group of closely related but distinguishable attitudes toward science and scientific methodology. Although by the 1930's most of the naturalistic viewpoint had lost its influence in America, parts of it survived. In particular, the faith of the naturalistic mind in "expertise"—in having trained persons in government—still exists in many quarters today. Since World War II other attitudes toward science have become popular and these also should not be confused with biological sociology. One is the view that science is essential both for national security and the American economy; the other is the faith that technology may solve problems of society (for example, by creating new pollution-cleaning devices as a means to combat the ecological crisis). Both ideas represent a type of application of science to society, but they are not what earlier writers had in mind when they spoke of society as organism and appealed to biology as a moral absolute to guide social behavior.

1930, extricating himself from what he considered an intolerable social situation. Upon arriving home, he was staggered by the lack of appreciation among his left-wing friends of the magnitude and danger of German race propaganda. His experiences in South Africa had convinced him that racism was internationally a fundamental issue—that what had happened in "the outpost of Empire" could also happen in "civilized" Europe. After accepting the newly created chair of Social Biology at the London School of Economics, which he was permitted to develop as he chose, he decided to try to put human genetics through a complete shake-up.[76] His writings on the subject thereafter castigated those who used the field as a takeoff for political speculation. He wrote in the preface to *Genetic Principles in Medicine and Social Science*:

Broadly speaking, the standpoint adopted [in this book] is that we can now entertain the prospect of fruitful development of human genetics as an exact science in close association with medicine, and it would, perhaps, be wiser to refrain from pretentious speculations concerning the relevance of genetic concepts to the study of human society until the subject has progressed considerably beyond its present boundaries.[77]

In *Nature and Nurture* he stressed that "it [human genetics] is not a panacea for human ailments"[78] and pointed out:

Human genetics is a very new department of scientific inquiry. In some quarters comprehensive claims have been put forward on its behalf. One school of opinion holds out the promise that a fuller understanding of the laws of human inheritance can disclose a clue to the rise and fall of civilisations. It is also urged that such knowledge can provide the only basis for a substantial improvement in the common lot of mankind. The grounds for such assertions are open to many criticisms.[79]

He proceeded to urge a more circumscribed but also more honorable role for the field:

Extravagant assurances of this kind do not alter the fact that human genetics has a genuine claim to be encouraged as a branch of medicine. The study of cancer has very little contribution to make to a scientific treatment of human history or to the removal of war, unemployment, and other evils which threaten the stability of existing civilisation. None the less it is a field of research which rightly engages the public esteem.[80]

76. Conversations with Lancelot Hogben, February 1–3, 1971.
77. Hogben, *Genetic Principles*, p. 9.
78. Hogben, *Nature and Nurture*, p. 10.
79. *Ibid.*, p. 9.
80. *Ibid.*, p. 9–10.

Others in this group agreed with Hogben. They too considered human genetics a science, not a justification of social behavior. Roberts felt very strongly about this point. He entered the field because it appealed to him as an intellectual exercise, just as if it were biochemistry. When Haldane demonstrated the linkage of hemophilia and color blindness in 1937, he was excited and impressed, even though there was no immediate social value to that discovery. He believed that one could think of the social implications of human genetics if one desired but that to do so was strictly extracurricular.[81] Crew recognized that the eugenic overtones of research in human genetics were hurting the field. He envisioned human genetics not as a political instrument but as a branch of medical science. In luncheon conversations with colleagues at the University of Edinburgh he advanced this position repeatedly.[82] Penrose also considered human genetics a part of medicine, and he expressed impatience with those who would use it to justify social policy. He complained:

A new science is liable to suffer from the premature popularization of the material with which it deals, and facts which have been ascertained with certainty may receive less consideration than tentative hypotheses. In the first enthusiasm the public may be misled into imagining that the laws which have been freshly discovered can at once have a wide application in the affairs of ordinary life.[83]

For taking such a stand he earned the enmity of E. J. Lidbetter, author of a book entitled *Heredity and the Social Problem Group*. During an interview arranged by the Eugenics Education Society, Lidbetter became so furious when Penrose disagreed with his view that pauperism is an inherited trait and that eugenic steps must be taken to solve the "problem" that he stormed away without even permitting Penrose to help him with his coat![84]

These men did not believe in biological sociology, and their rejection of this concept enabled them to possess a vision which many of the older geneticists did not have—a science of human genetics existing independently of eugenics. They did not deny human geneticists the right to their prejudices, but they did insist that the field did not exist to prove the social views of those who pursued it. They illustrated this outlook by deed as well as by word. Hogben, Haldane, and Penrose stood politically at the left; Fisher and Roberts at the right; yet they all approached the subject of

81. Conversation with Fraser Roberts, January 27, 1971.
82. Conversation with F. A. E. Crew, February 4, 1971.
83. Lionel Penrose, "Review of *Nature and Nurture*," *Politica*, 1(1934):225.
84. Conversation with Lionel Penrose, January 28, 1971.

human genetics the same way. Haldane, Muller, Hogben, and Fisher held controversial social opinions, including opinions about man's future genetic progress, but they still made brilliant scientific contributions—proof that human genetics could be approached objectively and critically, whatever the investigator's social views. In discussing applications of genetics, they distinguished between their roles as "scientists" (that is, explaining to the public the current state of knowledge) and their roles as "citizens" (that is, making moral judgments about the use of such knowledge) more frequently and more explicitly than most American geneticists, particularly the older ones.[85] This was a distinction which earlier writers on human genetics and eugenics did not make at all. The failure of earlier workers to do so is understandable in view of their conviction that biology should prescribe social behavior, but nonetheless it was a failure which made human genetics' association with eugenics a detrimental one for the science.

Curiously, these geneticists repudiated biological sociology at a time of great progress in the social sciences. At first glance it may seem that they did not recognize the advances in this area, but in fact they did. Professor Donald Fleming has pointed out that early sociologists from the time of Spencer believed that the task of the social sciences was to prescribe human conduct as well as to describe social phenomena. Statements by early eugenicists about the "religion of eugenics" fell into this tradition. Fleming feels that the social sciences became modern in the 1920's and 1930's because they *abandoned* their prescriptive duties.[86] In rejecting biological sociology these geneticists reacted to events in their science in a similar way. Unlike many of their predecessors, they refused to believe that the pursuit of biology would provide man moral and social guidance.

Thus, intellectual, historical, and sociological differences explained the respective attitudes of the American and English geneticists toward human genetics in the 1930's. The English workers pursued the field, despite their unhappiness with its eugenic overtones, because they approached genetic problems statistically, because eugenics had hindered human genetics less in England than in America, and because their rejection of biological sociology had enabled them to entertain the vision of human genetics as an independent science. They criticized earlier work in the field, but nevertheless they undertook the difficult task of upgrading the discipline's standards. Their efforts began the scientific reconstruction of the field.

85. See, for example, Haldane, *New Paths in Genetics*, pp. 35–36; and Hogben, *Genetic Principles*, p. 200.
86. Professor Donald Fleming, lectures on "The History of Science in America," Harvard University.

8

Reconstruction of Human Genetics

Though human genetics in America was at its low point in the 1930's, the field at that time began to be revitalized. During that decade a few persistent workers struggled successfully to keep the discipline alive. Impressed by their efforts, others began to pursue the subject, and human genetics began a slow growth which after World War II became self-sustaining. Progress in human genetics depended upon the infusion into the field of new, critical investigators, the development of sophisticated statistical and experimental techniques, and an increased appreciation of the science's applicability to medical problems. Yet social events, which had contributed to the field's decline, also contributed to its resurgence. In 1945, a critical period in the discipline's intellectual development, the widespread concern over the hazards of radiation which followed the sudden advent of the atomic age dramatically renewed interest in the subject. In the rhetoric of the 1970's, the field suddenly became "relevant," an event which did not cause its reconstruction but which certainly gave it impetus. The resurgence of human genetics therefore illustrated once again the interplay of scientific and non-scientific events in the field's development.

1. Scientific Advance

Throughout the Depression human genetics faced major problems. The field lacked funds, workers with critical acumen, and adequate training programs. Financial difficulties did not plague human genetics alone. Everywhere in genetics money was tight, and it was not uncommon for established investigators to have to perform routine tasks—preparing media and washing culture bottles—themselves. The economic situation of genetics was further complicated by the influx into the country of thousands of displaced European scholars, many of them biologists, searching for new positions in America at a time when openings in all areas were scarce. Nonetheless, conditions in human genetics were worse than in most specialties. Investigators trained in experimental genetics looked askance at a discipline where experimental methods seemed inapplicable. A cloud of opprobrium also hung over a field which some geneticists feared was oriented more toward politics than science.

In the 1930's and 1940's the situation in human genetics slowly began to change. Old-timers in human genetics passed away (Laughlin died in 1943, Davenport in 1944) and that style of worker in general was not replaced. A number of young men rigorously trained in experimental and statistical methods did not heed their seniors' warnings to stay away from human genetics and began working in the field. The last chapter already noted the efforts of Haldane, Fisher, Hogben, Roberts, and Penrose in England and Snyder and Muller (who wrote frequently on human genetics, though he experimented with Drosophila) in the United States. Of these men, Hogben was the chief apologist for human genetics. In addition to doing scientific work in the area, he enticed others into the field, most notably Haldane and Penrose. He and Haldane were close friends and agreeable rivals. They used to stay overnight at each other's houses, and they would pose problems for each other to solve. Before doing work in human genetics, Haldane had been interested mainly in biochemistry, but Hogben helped prod him into human genetics. Hogben would send Haldane reprints of everything he wrote, and he drew public attention to Haldane's work by discussing and interpreting it in his *Genetic Principles*.[1] Hogben also greatly stimulated Penrose's interest in the subject. In the 1930's the two held many conversations which reinforced Penrose's view that the study of mental deficiency offered an opportunity to perform important genetic research.[2]

A major influence upon the attitudes of the Englishmen toward human genetics was Archibald Garrod. All of them knew of his work on "inborn errors" and regarded it as an important contribution to human genetics, even though they did not yet recognize in it the "one-gene—one enzyme" concept. Haldane most frequently made public reference to Garrod, but Hogben was probably his keenest disciple. Hogben discovered Garrod's work while he was still in South Africa. He felt cheered by Garrod's investigations, seeing in them the first indication that human genetics had the potential to be developed into a valid science. Within six months after

1. Conversations with Lancelot Hogben, February 1–2, 1971.
2. Conversation with Lionel Penrose, January 25, 1971. Also, Lionel Penrose to author, October 13, 1970.

returning to England, Hogben made a special pilgrimage to Garrod's home, and later he returned for a second visit. They held long conversations about alkaptonuria, "inborn errors" in general, and the statistical analysis of pedigree data. Hogben was greatly influenced by these discussions, and shortly thereafter he performed a quantitative analysis of "familial diseases" in which he used the example of alkaptonuria.[3]

In America as well as England, talented new workers began to enter human genetics. In the mid-1930's Curt Stern, a distinguished experimentalist interested in chromosomal and developmental genetics, noticed the high percentage of pre-medical students in his undergraduate genetics course at the University of Rochester; for their benefit he included frequent references to human genetics. Soon afterwards he organized a graduate seminar on the subject, and thus began his career as one of this generation's eminent teachers and writers in the field.[4] A participant in that first seminar and later the first at Rochester to receive his Ph.D. (1939) from Stern—James V. Neel—was introduced to human genetics in the process.[5] In 1931 Clarence P. Oliver received a Ph.D. under H. J. Muller at the University of Texas for a project in radiation genetics. For two years thereafter he continued his research in basic genetics, studying gene nature, gene action, and causes of variability in genetic traits. When he went to the University of Minnesota in 1932, he began to work with the medical faculty and became interested in studying the genetics of man.[6] F. Clarke Fraser was a pre-medical candidate upon entering Acadia University in 1938, but he became enchanted with genetics while taking his freshman biology course. He pursued graduate studies in genetics at McGill, where he obtained a master's degree for a Drosophila cross-over problem and a Ph.D. for a developmental genetics problem in mice. He never relinquished his interest in medicine, however, and afterwards, with the encouragement of the chairman of his graduate department, C. L. Huskins, he entered medical school so that he could more effectively apply genetic techniques to medical problems.[7] While teaching introductory genetics at Harvard University, Sheldon Reed, a mouse and Drosophila geneticist, gradually came to recognize the importance of human genetics. In 1947 he switched over to the field, where he became especially interested in genetic counseling and the role of heredity in certain behavorial traits like mental retardation and the psychoses.[8] Individuals such as these

3. Conversation with Lancelot Hogben, February 2, 1971.
4. Conversation with Curt Stern, September 29, 1970.
5. *Ibid.* Neel later received an M.D. degree in 1944.
6. Clarence P. Oliver to author, August 4, 1970.
7. F. Clarke Fraser to author, August 25, 1970.
8. Sheldon Reed to author, July 28, 1970.

helped greatly to change opinion toward human genetics. The discipline no longer was a haven for dilettantes but was now being pursued by trained experimentalists who had passed through the scientific mill. A reviewer of Stern's *Principles of Human Genetics* (1949) could praise the author as "an accomplished Geneticist and distinguished research worker"[9] who is now writing on human genetics; such a compliment could seldom be given to earlier writers on the subject. The field thus grew in stature as the stature of the men who entered it increased.

At the same time the rate of advance in the subject started to accelerate. In the mid-1920's biologists began to recognize that the blood groups could be profitably studied with genetic techniques. From the start in 1900, investigation of the blood groups had proceeded entirely as a branch of medicine apart from both genetics and eugenics. Even in Germany this was so. In 1924, however, Felix Bernstein brought the blood groups into the province of human genetics by using the Hardy-Weinberg law to demonstrate that the ABO blood group system involves three genes rather than two as previously had been thought. Quickly thereafter the blood groups became the discipline's most important set of "test characters" for verifying theories of population genetics. In the 1930's major advances also occurred in the study of the inheritance of mental defectiveness. Prior to that time almost all work in mental deficiency had been alarmist, designed to spread the tale of the "menace of the feebleminded." Impressive pedigrees of degenerate families like the Jukes, the Nams, and the Dacks were invoked to impress upon the public the magnitude of the "problem." In the 1930's men such as Penrose and Roberts began to investigate the subject with sophisticated statistical techniques, thereby bringing the problem of mental defectiveness out of the hands of propagandists and amateur sociologists and into the province of medicine. Other advances followed. In 1937 Haldane discovered the first case of genetic linkage in man: the linkage of hemophilia and color blindness on the X-chromosome. In 1940 E. B. Ford of Oxford expounded the important concept of genetic polymorphism (the idea that non-pathological traits can occur in multiple forms, such as the ABO blood groups or the ability or the lack of ability to taste phenylthiocarbamide), a concept which has wide applications to all of genetics. In the 1930's many diseases, heretofore unsuspected of being hereditary, were demonstrated to follow Mendelian patterns of inheritance. Among the more famous of these were Tay-Sachs disease and phenylketonuria. In 1941 an important new category of genetic disease was discovered: materno-fetal incompatibility for the Rh blood group. In the preface to the 1946 edition of his book, Gates

9. E. B. Ford, "Review of *Principles of Human Heredity*," *Heredity*, 5(1951)153.

could rightly proclaim that "as in any rapidly developing field there are limitless opportunities for further research, but the time is now past when anyone can profitably suggest that little or nothing is known about heredity in man."[10]

These discoveries were important for more than purely intellectual reasons. They gave human genetics a start in medicine, which is an ideologically neutral field. Insofar as human genetics became part of medicine, it too became ideologically neutral, and this justified the faith of Hogben, Penrose, and others that human genetics could stand as an independent discipline apart from eugenics. The view that human genetics should be considered a part of medicine began to gain force in the 1930's, and it is significant that among the leading proponents of this position were many of those workers in human genetics, such as Hogben and Penrose, who were also critics of biological sociology and the use of human genetics to justify political theories. Hogben feels that perhaps the greatest contribution of persons like Penrose and Roberts, who are medical men, is their enormous influence in having human genetics become identified with medicine.[11] More shall be said on this matter later in the chapter.

As human genetics grew, institutional changes followed. The old Eugenics Record Office disappeared in 1940 when the Carnegie Institution hastened Laughlin's retirement and closed the office. This anachronism was replaced in the 1940's by modern centers of teaching and research in human genetics such as those at the Ohio State University, the University of Chicago, the University of Minnesota, the University of Michigan, the Bowman Gray School of Medicine, and the New York State Psychiatric Institute. The culminating events were the formation of the American Society of Human Genetics in 1948 and its journal, *The American Journal of Human Genetics*, in 1949. These last two occurrences marked the successful emergence of human genetics as an organized scientific discipline. It now boasted a society of its own, a regularly appearing publication to communicate research findings in the field, and departments and institutions which existed to promote research in the subject and to train future generations of investigators.

In the next two decades the field continued to expand. Between 1948 and 1970 the membership of the American Society of Human Genetics almost quadrupled,[12] and the number of workers in the field came to exceed greatly the membership of the society, as a perusal of the con-

10. R. Ruggles Gates, *Human Genetics*, vol. 1 (New York: Macmillan Co., 1946), p. vii.

11. Conversations with Lancelot Hogben, February 1–3, 1971.

12. Carl J. Witkop, Jr. to author, November 6, 1970. Dr. Witkop is secretary of the American Society of Human Genetics.

temporary literature attests. The subject has grown to such an extent that at present approximately a dozen journals in English regularly publish material on human genetics—a remarkable change from the earlier era in which not a single periodical was devoted exclusively to the subject. The number of departments, divisions, or sections of human or medical genetics in the United States has now risen to approximately seventy.[13] With the formation of a subsection on human genetics by the International Union of Biological Sciences and the holding of four highly successful international congresses of human genetics, international co-operation in the study of human inheritance has also increased.

During the last twenty years the study of human genetics has branched in many directions. The field has become so broad that one authority, Professor Victor McKusick of Johns Hopkins, now divides it into five main subspecialties: cytological and chromosomal genetics, biochemical genetics, immunogenetics, statistical and population genetics, and clinical genetics.[14] In all these areas major inroads have recently been achieved. Work has progressed rapidly in the study of human chromosome organization, gene localization, and genetic variation at the molecular level. Such investigations have been made possible by the development of powerful new experimental techniques like electron microscopy and tissue-culturing of human somatic cells. Biochemical studies of the structure of human proteins have yielded many inferences concerning the molecular mechanisms of gene action and evolution. A host of new "inborn errors" have been discovered, and in many cases the specific enzyme or chromosomal defect has also been identified. (The pioneering contributions of Archibald Garrod have indeed come to be appreciated!) The discovery of the human histocompatibility locus may result in applications to organ transplantation, and the further development and use of statistical techniques has enabled progress in the detection of genetic linkage in man and in the mapping of human chromosomes. Recent gains have also been made in the study of the genesis of congenital malformations.[15] Unlike the earlier era, when most investigators tended to view man primarily as an organism with which to test general principles derived from the study of other subjects, recent work in human genetics has yielded many results which are themselves of general importance. Perhaps the most fundamental such advance is the knowledge of gene action which has been derived from studies of

13. *Ibid.*
14. Victor A. McKusick, "Human Genetics," *Annual Review of Genetics*, 4(1970):1.
15. McKusick, *ibid.*, surveys the current scope and status of work in human genetics.

normal and aberrant human hemoglobin molecules. No longer is human genetics a topic for amateurs and dilettantes. Current methodology is exacting, and few pursue the subject today without a medical degree or a doctorate, which some now take in human genetics itself. The discipline has indeed become professionalized.

An indication of these changes was manifested in James Neel and William Schull's *Human Heredity* (1954), one of the important early postwar textbooks of the subject. The authors devoted their first chapter to dispelling views about research in human genetics which had not yet been destroyed. They decried the belief that human genetics still consisted simply of the collection of unusual pedigrees:

> Because of these shortcomings of human material, students of human heredity in the early decades of this century were for the most part led to confine their observations to the collection of extensive pedigrees in which a given trait appeared repeatedly in successive generations. There was a tendency to judge the value of the study in terms of the number of individuals in the pedigree. Under these circumstances the bulk of the attention was diverted to traits exhibiting simple dominant heredity. It was this early search for—and preoccupation with—families containing many persons affected with a given trait that has given rise to the belief, still encountered in some circles, that the study of human heredity consists in the collection of unusual, striking, and/or quaint pedigrees. As we shall see, this is far from the truth.[16]

They maintained that the study of human genetics could yield results of general significance, especially in the areas of biochemical and population genetics, which "are two subdivisions of genetics which are currently under intensive investigation [and] in which as much can be learned from the study of man as from any other animal."[17] They also stressed the importance to the discipline of proper methodology, particularly mathematical and statistical tools, warning the reader that the field had outgrown the stage in which undertrained, overly enthusiastic amateurs could reasonably hope to make meaningful contributions. "The reader who has not had college courses in the calculus and biometry may experience difficulty in places," they wrote. "We offer no apologies for this. The complexities of the study of human heredity are such that knowledge of certain branches of mathematics is no less essential to the serious student of human heredity than to the astronomer or the physical chemist. The

---

16. James V. Neel and William J. Schull, *Human Heredity* (Chicago: The University of Chicago Press, 1954), pp. 1–2.
   17. *Ibid.*, p. 2.

text which attempts to disguise this fact is, in the long run, doing the student a disservice."[18]

Since the war, human genetics has earned the praise of leading geneticists. Participants at the Eighth and Ninth International Congresses of Genetics (Stockholm, 1948, and Bellagio, 1953) first suggested that an international congress of human genetics would be worthwhile.[19] Professor J. W. Boyes, President of the Genetics Section of the International Union of Biological Sciences, told the Second International Congress of Human Genetics (Rome, 1961):

> I can assure you from my personal experience that recent progress in Genetics and particularly in Human Genetics is most impressive. . . . We all know that Human Genetics has matured and grown greatly in its scope and value in recent years. This is amply demonstrated by the presence here of so many eager participants. All geneticists are delighted with your progress and increasing stature.[20]

At the same meeting Nobel laureate Edward L. Tatum declared: "The past decade has seen tremendous and exciting developments in the vast and important area of Human Genetics. The scope of this most timely conference is ample evidence of the increasing recognition of the potentialities of studies on the human organism both in furthering our basic knowledge of gene action and in the application of this knowledge."[21] Nobel Prize winner George Beadle remarked to the Third International Congress of Human Genetics in 1966: "It is gratifying to know that within the past two decades human genetics has really come into its own. . . . Here we are today, reviewing the truly remarkable progress that has been made on multiple fronts."[22] Such words perhaps stand as the most significant testimony to the "arrival" of human genetics. Whereas earlier experimental geneticists grew to distrust the field, leading experimentalists of the present now commend it. Workers in human genetics have succeeded in winning the critical acclaim of those whose respect they most needed.

Despite their successes, many workers in human genetics in one respect are still cautious about the future. Recognizing the social implications of some of their work, they are fearful lest anyone again pervert the subject for political or private purposes. This apprehension was particularly

18. *Ibid.*, p. 4.

19. Luida Gedda, "Historical Retrospect," in *Proceedings of the Second International Congress of Human Genetics*, vol. 1 (Rome: Istituto G. Mendel, 1963), p. 46*.

20. Untitled address of Professor J. W. Boyes, *ibid.*, vol. 1, p. 82*.

21. Edward L. Tatum, "Microbial and Biochemical Genetics," *ibid.*, vol. 1, p. 509.

22. George W. Beadle, "Welcoming Address," in *Proceedings of the Third International Congress of Human Genetics* (Baltimore: Johns Hopkins Press, 1967), p. 3.

noticeable during the first few years following the formation of the American Society of Human Genetics. Many at that time reiterated their *scientific* interest in the subject and exposed those who failed to approach the subject sufficiently objectively and disinterestedly. In his presidential address to the society in 1952, Franz J. Kallmann declared, "No redundance is necessary in acknowledging the truism that a strictly scientific search for the facts and potential implications of human heredity will always be our chief objective."[23] He described how "the spirit which prevailed in this Society during the first few years of its existence gravitated in the direction of intellectual individualism mixed with pronounced caution."[24] In his presidential address to the society ten years later, F. Clarke Fraser stated:

I don't want to detract at all from the impressive accomplishments I have already mentioned. But let us not oversell ourselves, and let us protect the prestige of Human Genetics from jeopardy by unqualified people speaking irresponsibly in its name. It happened before, and it could happen again. Much genetic nonsense is still being written about race (e.g., Putnam, 1961), people are still getting data to fit Mendelian ratios by such errors as omitting to omit the proband, and still invoking reduced penetrance and other euphemisms for ignorance to account for deviations from Mendelian expectations that can better be accounted for by other mechanisms.[25]

These examples are not intended to suggest that present-day investigators in human genetics are uninterested in eugenic or social applications of the science, for many find such applications desirable. Kallman himself remained active in the American Eugenics Society until his death in 1966. Nevertheless, most of these men, whether interested in social applications of their work or not, distinguish between research in human genetics and applications thereof, and they demand that any application be critically considered from both a scientific and ethical point of view.

In the 1940's, therefore, human genetics overcame its slow start and began growing at a rate which finally became self-sustaining. The tempo of research quickened even more in the 1950's and 1960's as workers made many discoveries of far-reaching importance. Human genetics at present is by no means pre-eminent among the biological sciences, but unquestionably it has gained recognition as a rigorous, intellectually respectable

23. Franz J. Kallmann, "Human Genetics as a Science, as a Profession, and as a Social-Minded Trend of Orientation," *American Journal of Human Genetics*, 4(1952):241.
24. *Ibid.*, p. 239.
25. F. Clarke Fraser, "On Being a Medical Geneticist," *American Journal of Human Genetics*, 15(1963):2.

field. An editorial in the *American Journal of Human Genetics* marking the arrival of the 1970's could correctly proclaim: "Human genetics has grown considerably since the *Journal* first appeared in 1949. Few areas of human biology have remained untouched by this evolving field; its implications for medicine have become particularly apparent, and genetic research related to man is now vigorously pursued in many medical schools."[26] The future prospects for human genetics are indeed bright.

2. The "New Eugenics"

While new workers began to rebuild human genetics in the 1930's, analogous events were occurring within the American eugenics movement. By the middle of the decade the "old" eugenics movement had collapsed. Undaunted by its failure, a new leadership, genuinely interested in mankind's genetic future, assumed the task of rebuilding it. They rejected the class and race biases of their predecessors, admitted the foolishness of earlier eugenicists' biological pronouncements, and propounded a new eugenics creed which was both scientifically and philosophically attuned to a changed America.

The reconstruction began in 1928 when Frederick Osborn, who was to become the driving force of a revitalized eugenics, made his sudden and unexpected entrance into the movement. Though he had embarked on a highly successful business career (he had been a railroad president, a director of several corporations, and a partner in a banking firm), he also had been interested in evolution, man, and anthropology since 1908, when he had taken a course at Princeton under William Scott, professor of geology and biology. In 1928, at age forty, he retired from business and threw himself into the eugenics movement. In a short while he had become treasurer of the American Eugenics Society and one of the movement's leading spokesmen. At that time he also launched an intensive reading campaign into the latest literature of genetics, psychology, sociology, and anthropology which convinced him that the broad generalizations commonly promulgated by eugenicists were unsound. As men like Grant and Laughlin passed away, he used his influence to ensure that they were replaced as officers of eugenic organizations by individuals of more balanced views.[27]

26. Arno G. Motulsky, "Editorial: *The American Journal of Human Genetics* in the 1970's," *American Journal of Human Genetics*, 22(1970):109.

27. Frederick Osborn to author, November 5, 1970; and Mark H. Haller, *Eugenics: Hereditarian Attitudes in American Thought* (New Brunswick, New Jersey: Rutgers University Press, 1963), pp. 174–75.

In the 1930's individuals like Osborn gradually developed a new eugenics philosophy, one which was much less dogmatic and considerably more modest in tone. Unlike previous eugenicists they did not entreat for legislation but quietly encouraged research in human genetics, demography, psychology, and anthropology. Criticizing earlier treatments of the subject, they conceded environmental influences to be as important in human development as genes. Osborn wrote, "Belief in the influence of heredity over-reached itself when it was used—as it still is all too often—to justify the continued domination of some particular caste or group."[28] F. Stuart Chapin observed:

Fortunately for those who advocate a positive emphasis upon the preservation of sound human stock, the eugenics movement of the past two decades has sloughed off its earlier overemphasis upon pure genetics and oriented itself to the findings of increasingly discriminating research on environmental factors. Consequently the eugenics movement is today implemented by a rapidly accumulating knowledge derived from experimental and statistical research on the relationship of man to his present environment.[29]

These men recognized the importance of favorable public opinion to a successful eugenics program, and accordingly they insisted that leadership of the movement be intelligent, balanced, non-controversial.

At a time when the majority of Americans were growing suspicious of the spectre of fascism, the new spokesmen also repudiated the class and race biases which had been dominating the movement as well as the movement's insistence upon compulsory sterilization laws. They declared that a "true" eugenics program is possible only in a democratic framework where the right to have children is protected and where eugenic programs would supplement all other efforts at social advance and environmental reform. Such a program, they maintained, would allow for many types of individuals and cultures. In a very important passage Osborn wrote:

Eugenics and democracy are significantly interrelated. The eugenics ideal calls for a society so organized that eugenic selection will take place as a natural and largely unconscious process; one in which those persons who make the most effective response to their environment will, in the normal course, have more children than those who respond less effectively. That kind of eugenics would be the only kind possible in a democracy where, except in cases of extreme defect, no one would be given or would assume any right to decide who should or who should not have children.

28. Frederick H. Osborn, *Preface to Eugenics* (New York: Harper and Brothers, 1940), p. 42.
29. F. Stuart Chapin, "Editor's Introduction," *ibid.*, p. vii.

The right to have or not to have children would be safeguarded in a democracy along with the right to free speech and to freedom of worship. This is a necessary protection to eugenics, for man himself is not fitted to judge right and wrong so clearly that broad power over survival would be safe in any hands except those of the parents who are directly concerned. Only in a dictatorship would such power be taken from the mass of parents and put under arbitrary control. A system of arbitrary control would not be eugenics, but would be simply the application of genetic science to the breeding of specific kinds of men and women. This is something which could easily be done. It would be as dangerous as putting any other tools of modern science in the hands of arbitrary power.[30]

This revamped eugenics credo was advanced most fully in Osborn's *Preface to Eugenics*, a book which remains even today the standard text of the American eugenics movement.[31]

By the late 1930's the transformation within the eugenics movement had become apparent. At the 1932 International Eugenics Congress in New York, Robert Cook correctly sensed the impending demise of old-style eugenics, lamenting: "Until a Eugenics Congress is at least as well attended as a political convention, we have failed of our mission. If, with all the compelling arguments and really fascinating facts at our command, we cannot bring this about we must, I fear, concede that the popular writers are right, and that we rightly deserve the approbrious [sic!] title 'half-baked'!"[32] Shortly thereafter institutional changes within the movement began. In 1939 the *Journal of Heredity*, previously an outlet for much uncritical writing on eugenic matters, announced a new policy toward the subject. An editorial proclaimed: "The revolution in eugenic thinking which has been taking place might be appropriately labeled 'The Democratic Approach to Eugenics.' The original Galtonian eugenics was distinctly an affair of a chosen class and of a chosen nation even."[33] The American Eugenics Society in 1937 still said of its goals as a society: "It [the society] also advocates such measures as selective immigration, the sterilization or segregation of hereditary defectives, and the spread of birth control in order to reduce the size of families among parents who are unable rightly to train their children."[34] In 1942 it announced a new purpose: "to maintain an educational membership society consisting of

30. Osborn, *Preface to Eugenics*, pp. 297–98.
31. For a shorter statement of the new credo, see Frederick H. Osborn, "Development of a Eugenic Philosophy," *American Sociological Review*, 2(1937):389.
32. Robert Cook, "Is Eugenics Half-Baked?" in *A Decade of Progress in Eugenics* (Baltimore: Williams and Wilkins Co., 1934), p. 446.
33. Editor, "A Quarterly Eugenics Section," *Journal of Heredity*, 30(1939):108.
34. *Scientific and Technical Societies and Institutions of the United States and Canada*, 3rd ed. (Washington, D.C.: National Research Council–National Academy of Sciences, 1937), p. 34.

and directed by scientists, professionals, and laymen who are interested in public welfare generally, and specifically in interpreting the development of a sound democratic program for improving the quality of the American people."[35] Osborn firmly refused back issues of the *Eugenical News* for the files of the American Eugenics Society when they were offered to him.[36] A new journal, *Eugenics Quarterly*, declared in its opening editorial in 1954:

> The public has first to learn that race and social classes are relatively of little importance as indices of hereditary capacity. This is not an easy lesson to learn. We all like to think that our own group of people has superior qualities. . . . It should be the most immediate task of eugenics to substitute for this ancient form of self-admiration the knowledge that hereditary capacities are widely scattered throughout the human race, among families within every social class and within every geographic area. This is the message of science.[37]

The editorial proceeded to advance reasons "why eugenics can only succeed in a democracy."[38]

Since World War II the reconstructed eugenics movement has succeeded in gaining the scientific respect of most geneticists, regardless of their individual moral views about eugenic programs. One sign of its newly found scientific acceptance is that leading biologists, such as Joshua Lederberg and, in later life, H. J. Muller, have once again become leading proponents of eugenic schemes.[39] During the past twenty-five years the American Eugenics Society has benefited from the involvement of many prominent scientists on its board of directors. Since the board now consists of approximately twenty-five members, compared to over one hundred before the Depression, the scientists' influence is relatively undiluted. In recent years eugenic societies have sponsored studies and symposia which have received critical acclaim from other biologists. It was significant when a reviewer of a 1964 Eugenics Society conference wrote in *Heredity*: "It must be made clear that the papers themselves are of a high standard and well worth possessing. The reviewer found many of the

35. *Ibid.*, 4th ed., p. 45.
36. Haller, *Eugenics*, p. 180.
37. "The Role of the American Eugenics Society," *Eugenics Quarterly*, 1(1954):2.
38. *Ibid.*, p. 3.
39. In *Out of the Night* (New York: Vanguard Press, 1935), Muller suggested applying artificial insemination to man for eugenic purposes, and he remained the leading proponent of this procedure until his death in 1967. His was a very idiosyncratic approach to eugenics. At once he was a leftist, an anti-racist, and a harsh critic of the earlier eugenics movement as well as a leading proponent of artificial insemination and genetic uplift.

papers quite fascinating. . . . This collection of papers is an important contribution to our understanding of the biology of man."[40] So scientifically oriented have certain eugenic societies become today that some believe they have lost sight of their original purpose of promoting genetic uplift! In 1969 the *Eugenics Review* changed its title to the *Journal of Biosocial Science.* Most biologists probably would agree with James Crow, a population geneticist at the University of Wisconsin, who remarked: "I distinguish, of course, between a scientifically competent, socially thoughtful study of ways of genetic improvement of mankind—not the perversions of Nazi Germany or the simplification, and occasional downright foolishness of the early American eugenics movement."[41]

Apart from the encouragement of research (the American Eugenics Society, for example, co-sponsored the United States National Committee to the First International Congress of Human Genetics and since then has supported much important work in clinical genetics and demography), the eugenics program of today has two main parts. The first and less controversial is genetic counseling, the advising of prospective parents of the probability that their children will be born with a genetic condition, a service which many medical institutions already provide. Most genetic counselors do not consider themselves eugenicists; still, the eugenic overtones of their work are obvious, and heredity clinics are endorsed by most of those who do advocate eugenic measures. Stern has pointed out that "genetic counseling is largely devoted to individual problems, although the social implications of any specific advice usually are not disregarded."[42] In his textbook he used the term "genetic counseling" interchangeably with "eugenic counseling."[43] C. Nash Herndon, a pioneer in medical genetics and genetic counseling, wrote: "The counselor concerned with any problem of heredity must always bear in mind the possible eugenic or dysgenic effect of any advice he may give. The counselor must not only be concerned with the specific problem in inheritance raised by a given family but must also attempt to make some assay of the total genetic endowment of the persons in question."[44] Through the years, developments in genetic counseling have been sympathetically followed in such periodicals as the *Eugenics Quarterly.*

40. P. M. Sheppard, "Review of *Biological Aspects of Social Problems,*" *Heredity*, 22(1967):311.

41. James Crow to author, July 29, 1970.

42. Curt Stern, *Principles of Human Genetics*, 2nd ed. (San Francisco: W. H. Freeman and Company, 1960), p. 665.

43. *Ibid.*, pp. 665–66.

44. C. Nash Herndon, "Heredity Counseling," *Eugenics Quarterly*, 2(1955):88–89.

The second and more controversial part, sometimes itself referred to as the "new eugenics," is the dramatic new vision of man's future brought about by post-war advances in molecular biology. With the structure and principal mechanisms of the gene having been elucidated, bold visionaries predict and in some cases anticipate a day when physicians will dispense test-tube babies and prevent hereditary conditions by genetic surgery! Sometimes the new eugenics goes by the name "genetic engineering," though in actuality it encompasses more than just genetic surgery as that name implies. Strictly speaking it may involve environmental manipulation; nonetheless it represents the utilization of genetic techniques. However bizarre and science-fiction-sounding genetic engineering may seem, in certain ways it also resembles the less imaginative eugenic programs of the past. Now, as before, the major controversy surrounding eugenics is one of ethics and not of science, of means and not of ends. Furthermore, most present-day eugenicists discuss genetic engineering mainly as a potential cure for various "inborn errors of metabolism"; like their predecessors in the eugenics movement they are speaking of conditions caused by single genes. In this particular respect, modern advocates of genetic engineering are today's equivalent to the early Mendelians.

Though a great ethical controversy surrounds it, the idea of genetic engineering has arisen from brilliant scientific work—indeed, from Nobel Prize winning discoveries. For the future of genetic engineering this is, I think, a danger as well as a strength. The hazard is that enthusiasts of genetic engineering may be approaching the subject too objectively, too scientifically. Many are convinced that man's understanding of genetics far exceeds his wisdom to apply that knowledge ethically and beneficially. Some fear that proponents of genetic engineering regard it so much as an intellectual problem that they neglect to consider its effects on the individual and society. One well-known investigator has urged: "If this investigation [work in genetic engineering] is done with man, the study should be made with collaborators who can protect genetics from public scorn by having scientists working with articulate sociologists and psychologists who plan for a long time before doing the engineering."[45] Thus, modern eugenicists have performed an about-face from an earlier era in which their predecessors were reproached for *not* being objective enough in pursuing the genetics of man.

It is not surprising that some enthusiasts have been accused of approaching genetic engineering too objectively. Genetic engineering is in fact a genetic technology, and as a form of technology it suffers from the

45. Clarence P. Oliver to author, August 4, 1970.

same problem of "technology without a 'logos' " that Herbert Marcuse has described for other forms of technology. Marcuse has discussed the tendency for science and technology to become the instrumentalities of "experts" who are so interested in "making it work" that they neglect to ask the value questions "for what?" and "for whom?"[46] Engineers might come to consider "building the perfect bridge" an end in itself, not caring whether a bridge in a certain site is needed; surgeons might become obsessed with the idea of "the perfect operation" or "the perfect transplant," forgetting that medicine's task is "to save lives." It thus becomes understandable why the tendency to some is so great to treat genetic engineering wholly as a scientific matter—this is the manifestation of a general dilemma affecting much of the rest of technology as well.

Another dilemma surrounds genetic engineering, a general one which faces all of American society: the problem of differentiating problems of "technique" from problems of "value." Since the second World War science and technology have played such important roles in American affairs that for a while many regarded them (and some still do) as "cure-alls" for any problem. Recently it has been recognized increasingly that not all problems can be solved by technique and expertise—that underneath certain apparent questions of methodology and technology lie questions of value. It has been suggested, for example, that the solution to the ecological crisis does not depend solely upon the development of better laws and more sophisticated equipment to clean pollution, but also upon making a fundamental ethical and moral conversion to the view that saving the environment is an imperative—a switch analogous to the moral conversion abolitionists made in relinquishing slave ownership as a "natural property right" of man.[47] Laws and equipment are necessary to resolve the ecological crisis, but so also is the re-examination of underlying political and philosophical beliefs, such as whether air and water are free commodities and whether land and its resources may be used in accordance with the unrestricted desires of their private owners.[48] In discussing the use of any science, including genetics, to solve social problems, it therefore becomes important to demarcate clearly the *limit* that scientific technique may be expected to contribute to an effective solution. Small wonder,

46. Herbert Marcuse, *One-Dimensional Man; Studies in the Ideology of Advanced Industrial Society* (Boston: Beacon Press, 1964).
47. James Reston, "The Ethics of the Land," Baltimore *Evening Sun*, August 10, 1970, p. A-10.
48. James Reston, "Humans vs. Property," Baltimore *Evening Sun*, August 31, 1970, p. A-8. See also James Reston, "Even the Philosophers are at Bay," Baltimore *Evening Sun*, September 2, 1970, p. A-14.

then, that the debate over genetic engineering has been so muddled and confused.

Following the example of earlier geneticists who exercised their "social responsibility," many current workers in genetics and human genetics have attempted to guide the public discussion of eugenics. They believe, as Dunn remarked in 1962, that "the social and political misuse to which genetics applied to man is peculiarly subject is influenced not only by those who support such misuse, but also by those who fail to point out, as teachers, the distinctions between true and false science."[49] Like earlier geneticists, they also have recognized that biologists operate in a social context, that all scientists are products of their personal histories, that biologists act as both "scientists" and "citizens."[50] Such efforts have been beneficial, but unresolved problems still remain. Despite geneticists' attempts to evoke widespread discussion of genetic engineering, the public

49. L. C. Dunn, "Cross Currents in the History of Human Genetics," *American Journal of Human Genetics*, 14(1962):8.
This discussion should not be interpreted to imply that a majority, or even a significant percentage, of geneticists are actively carrying out their "social responsibility." In fact, scientists traditionally have tended to abstain from political or social involvement of any sort; there has always been an undercurrent of suspicion toward anyone who would dare venture from the laboratory into the world of popular writing or speaking. Hogben prefaced his *Science for the Citizen* by assuring the readers, especially the scientists among them, that he had not sacrificed "working time" to write the book since he had written it during spare moments on railroad trips! Today, however, with science such a major part of the gross national product, with technology rapidly altering the mode of human existence, traditional resistance to a scientist's social or political involvement—at least in matters relating directly to the financing or application of science—is slowly breaking down. A "socially concerned" community of scientists implies that the leaders of the field are authorized to speak for the group, not that greater than fifty percent are letter writers and banner carriers. The International Congresses of Human Genetics of 1956 and 1961 passed resolutions, for example, and afterwards, as the delegates returned to the laboratory, the officers of the Congresses publicized the resolutions as "representatives of human genetics." Only a few men acted as publicists, but they represented the views of many.
50. The 1960's witnessed many symposiums on the genetic future of man, and in most of these various participants distinguished between a technical understanding of genetics and the ethical wisdom with which to use it. In one such symposium Polykarp Kusch stated: "Nothing is more destructive of rational thought about science-related problems than the common belief that everything a scientist says is validated by the criteria of formal science. We are all products of our personal history and that of our society." Polykarp Kusch, "Introductory Statement," in John D. Roslansky, ed., *Genetics and the Future of Man* (New York: Appleton-Century-Crofts, 1966), pp. 5–6. For other examples see Tracy M. Sonneborn, "Preface," in Sonneborn, ed., *The Control of Human Heredity and Evolution* (New York: The Macmillan Company, 1965), pp. viii–ix; and "Social and Cultural Evolution," Panel Five, in Sol Tax and Charles Callender, eds., *Evolution After Darwin*, vol. 3 (Chicago: The University of Chicago Press, 1960), pp. 240–41.

often seems more inclined to accede to the views of the authorities than to debate the issue. The tendency is very great indeed to assume that a man with the technical knowledge of a field is somehow more qualified to pass judgment on its applications, even if he claims he is speaking "only as a citizen." Today, when mass media enables the opinions of the famous to be heard everywhere, this tendency may even be accentuated. A famous biologist might describe his "view of the future" on one of the network television "talk shows" before millions of home viewers; even if he is alarmed by that view, he runs the danger of being thought to condone it and thereby of unintentionally helping to bring it about. Statements on genetic engineering carry the risk of becoming self-fulfilling prophesies.

In the last three decades, the eugenics movement, like the science of human genetics, has undergone its scientific reconstruction. Although opinion varies greatly regarding the technical feasibility, morality, and need of eugenic measures, the scientific work which has stimulated recent eugenic speculation is sound. The topic of genetic engineering has engendered an especially great controversy, but this controversy embraces more than the issue of genetic engineering alone, since it involves fundamental ethical and philosophical questions which also underlie many other perplexing issues facing contemporary America.

3. Medicine and Genetics

In the 1930's the American medical profession began to display a more receptive attitude toward genetics and human genetics. New in that decade was not a sudden interest in heredity among physicians but rather the emergence of the concept that human genetics is a branch of medical research. Many physicians at that time started to show greater interest in hereditary diseases, and some began to urge that genetics be included in the medical curriculum. For human genetics this change in attitude occurred at an opportune moment since it justified the claim of men like Hogben that the discipline could contribute to medical science. As human genetics came to be identified with medicine, it was increasingly recognized to be a legitimate scientific field. Acceptance of the idea of medical genetics came slowly and with difficulty, but by the early 1950's clinical genetics had clearly entered American medicine and was preparing to undergo a very rapid burst of progress. The new association between medicine and genetics was to prove highly profitable to both.

At the start of the Depression, American medicine paid scarcely more attention to genetics than it had for the preceding three decades. Almost every American medical school failed to provide formal instruction in genetics. The most instruction that students usually received in the subject consisted of sporadic asides by heredity-minded clinicians at the bedside or a few perfunctory lectures included somewhere in the course of study. Macklin complained in 1932: "This knowledge [heredity of disease], it is true, has not been taught to the medical student in the past, except as it came in as an aside in the clinical lectures of some clinician particularly interested in heredity.... The students of today are receiving little information on the subject and as they become the clinical teachers of tomorrow, the lack of teaching in this branch will continue."[51] Some physicians did publish their clinical observations on the inheritance of various diseases, but they were far outnumbered by physicians who were skeptical of the role of heredity in disease and who considered their own personal observations of conditions running in families to be "insufficiently important" to report in the clinical literature.[52] Physicians did show a small amount of interest in "inborn errors of metabolism"—Osler's textbook of medicine from the sixth edition (1905) onward mentioned Garrod's work on alkaptonuria—but the prevailing view among medical men was that these diseases were merely academic playthings of no social or practical importance. These conditions occurred so very rarely that most physicians would spend their entire careers without even seeing a single case.

As the 1930's opened, however, the practice of medicine had been undergoing certain changes which gradually had made it more receptive to the idea that parts of genetic science fall into its domain. First, by 1930 many traditional killers among infectious diseases had been conquered owing to the rise of bacteriology as an exact science and the beginning of the age of chemotherapy. Many diseases of malnutrition had likewise been defeated. Between 1900 and 1930 the average life expectancy had increased from forty-eight to sixty. Many individuals who previously might have succumbed to infection were now seeing their physicians because of constitutional disorders such as diabetes, cancer, stroke, and heart disease,

51. Madge Thurlow Macklin, "The Teaching of Inheritance of Disease," *Annals of Internal Medicine*, 6(1933):1336.

52. Macklin provided the following example of the skepticism toward the role of heredity in disease of some physicians she had encountered: "At a recent talk before physicians, I was astonished to find the numerous striking instances of pathological conditions which even a group of only twenty-five men could recall from their practices. In some cases the knowledge of the condition in other members of the family was of help in diagnosis. Thus they recalled a parent and two children with heart block; a man and his son operated upon for renal calculi; three generations of displaced lens; marked mental deficiency in mother and children; pernicious anemia running through several generations, etc. But none of these had ever crept into the clinical literature, because they had not seemed of sufficient importance. Yet we have those who are skeptical of the influence of heredity in disease, because there are so few published records of it." *Ibid.*, pp. 1336–37.

many of which were seen to have a hereditary background. Because people were living longer, individuals afflicted with late-onset hereditary conditions like pernicious anemia developed symptoms of the full disease more and more frequently. The practicing physician could not escape the realization that he would now increasingly confront diseases of genetic as well as environmental etiology. Medical school curriculum committees could no longer so facilely argue that by including instruction in genetics they would be adding material to an already overcrowded teaching schedule which the future practicing physician would not use.

Second, the philosophical base of medicine had broadened to include the concept of prevention. The first three decades of the century were as much a time of improved sanitation and of innovative public health measures as they were of new methods to treat infection, and in the 1930's the idea of preventive medicine gained a still stronger foothold. The application of genetic principles to medical problems harmonized exceedingly well with this philosophical shift. With a knowledge of heredity, the physician could advise prospective parents afflicted with genetic conditions and thereby prevent the unwitting passage of a disease to subsequent generations. Such knowledge would also arm him with a high index of suspicion when examining relatives of individuals with a genetically-determined condition; he would be alerted to watch for early symptoms of the same disease so that if necessary he could rapidly begin appropriate treatment.

Lastly, the tools of human genetics had become sufficiently developed by the 1930's that they could be applied to certain medical problems. Prior to 1930, despite the sparsity of knowledge in the field, some of the data that were available could still be utilized by physicians. Studies of human genetics mainly had consisted of attempts to discover the patterns of inheritance of various pathological conditions—precisely the information that physicians most needed in their practices. By this time the application of the population and statistical approach to humans also had reaped certain dividends for medical genetics, particularly knowledge of the blood groups. The discovery of the Rhesus antigen (the "Rh factor") in 1941 brought the blood groups into still greater prominence; there could be no doubt about the significance of genetics for medicine in this important clinical situation. In the 1930's, moreover, a number of new genetic diseases were discovered, including phenylketonuria, the first "inborn error" which was not exceedingly rare.[53]

Amidst these changes began the campaign to place genetics in the American medical curriculum. Pioneers in this struggle were Laurence

53. Penrose points out that Hitler's scientists did not accept phenylketonuria because of its frequent occurrence in Aryan stocks of Norway. They did not believe

Snyder, Madge Thurlow Macklin, and William Allan. Snyder, a Ph.D., had obtained his degree under William Castle at Harvard, having written his dissertation on the inheritance of the human blood groups. Macklin and Allan were medical doctors. Throughout the 1930's and into the 1940's, in speeches, symposia, meetings, and papers, they urged repeatedly that genetics be added to the medical curriculum. They argued that a knowledge of genetics would increase the physician's theoretical understanding of disease and aid him in the practical areas of diagnosis, therapy, prognosis, and prevention. With an increased number of record gatherers, they predicted that genetics too would benefit from such an association. All three, but particularly Macklin, advanced this position with missionary zeal. They argued theoretically; they also provided numerous examples to illustrate concretely how an understanding of genetics could serve the physician. Instance after instance was given to counteract the view that nothing practical was known about human genetics and to reinforce their position that such knowledge could be of value in the everyday practice of medicine.

During the 1930's and 1940's these ideas gradually came to be accepted. In 1933 Ohio State, where Snyder was working, became the first to institute a required course in medical genetics. After this initial success, American medicine began to become more receptive to hereditarian notions, though changes occurred very slowly. In 1940 Amram Scheinfeld, a popularizer of genetic science and an astute observer of the status of the field, could still justifiably lament:

It seems surprising that so few medical men are aware of the possibilities which the increasing store of knowledge in this field [human genetics] holds for them. . . . Even today medical genetics, as a special subject, has not yet found its way into the curricula of more than two or three medical colleges in this country. . . . While the United States has led the world in experimental genetics, we have allowed the initiative in medical genetics to be taken by a number of other countries (notably Germany, where unfortunately, some aspects of the science are being distorted toward questionable ends).[54]

Nevertheless, the gains which accrued were permanent. The cause of medical genetics was aided by the aforementioned discovery of the Rh factor in 1941 as well as by the publication the year before of an influ-

---

there could be an "Aryan disease." Earlier these scientists had accepted amaurotic idiocy (Tay-Sachs disease), which has a high incidence in Ashkenazic Jews, because they considered it a "Jewish disease." (Conversation with Lionel Penrose, January 28, 1971.)

54. Amram Scheinfeld, "Genetics and the Medical Man," *Human Fertility*, 5(1940):129.

ential series of guest lectures in medical genetics that Snyder had given at the Duke University School of Medicine. A survey in 1946 showed that 38 per cent of American medical schools assigned some time to the teaching of genetics, including seven schools which offered formal courses in the subject;[55] a similar survey in 1953 showed that 55 per cent of the medical schools in the country included instruction in genetics.[56] American medicine, at least at the academic level, had finally become more cordial to genetics, and the stage was set for the "takeoff" in medical genetics of the late 1950's.[57]

The pioneering efforts in the 1930's to introduce the teaching of genetics to American medical students were significant for still another reason: those who led the campaign were motivated partly by a "eugenic impulse." Allan entitled one of his articles "Medicine's Need of Eugenics."[58] Snyder, who earlier had served on the publications committee of the Third International Eugenics Congress in 1932, felt that one reason genetic knowledge could be of use to physicians is that "it may provide the necessary information for setting up eugenic and euthenic programs for the protection of society, in which every physician should be able to take an intelligent part, based upon experimental data, not opinion, prejudice, and overexaggerating the uncertainties."[59] Later he became a member of the Board of Directors of the American Eugenics Society. Addressing the Third International Eugenics Congress, Macklin claimed that the addition of genetics to the medical curriculum is "a pivotal point in the eugenic program."[60] "A sound eugenic measure," she declared, "and one which

55. G. G. Robertson and J. C. Haley, "Genetics in the Medical Curriculum," *Journal of the Association of American Medical Colleges*, 21(1946):352.

56. C. Nash Herndon, "Human Genetics and Medical Education," *Journal of Medical Education,* 29/7 (1954): 14–15.

57. In England, too, efforts began in the 1930's to have genetics taught to medical students, though that country has lagged behind America in doing so. Hogben, Penrose, Haldane, and Roberts frequently lamented the omission of genetics from the English medical curriculum and urged that it be instated. During his career Hogben has been associated with three medical schools, and at each he worked hard to have genetics added as a course. He succeeded at Capetown and Aberdeen, failed at Birmingham. (He was at Birmingham at a time when the medical schools were transferring much of the teaching of preliminary biology to an earlier stage of education in order to make more room for returning World War II veterans.) With regard to the teaching of fundamental biology to medical students, he considers himself a "missionary of American culture" to British medical education, and his own courses always stressed an integrative approach to basic biology. (Conversations with Lancelot Hogben, February 1–3, 1971.)

58. William Allan, "Medicine's Need of Eugenics," *Southern Medicine and Surgery*, 98(1936):416.

59. Laurence Snyder, *Medical Genetics* (Durham, N. C.: Duke University Press, 1940), pp. 3–4.

60. Madge Macklin, "The Need of a Course in Medical Genetics in the Medical Curriculum," in *A Decade of Progress in Eugenics*, p. 157.

will bring in large returns in professional and public interest, and which will serve to give far more data on human inheritance than we have at present, is the agitation to have taught in every medical school, not only a more extensive course of the fundamentals of genetics in pre-medical courses, but the application of this science to problems of human disease."[61] Others also espoused this view. In a speech before the forty-second annual meeting of the Association of American Medical Colleges in 1931, E. P. Lyon, dean of the University of Minnesota Medical School, stated: "I think heredity has a close relation to medicine—an increasingly important relation. I think doctors will have to be leaders in any effective program of eugenics or of the use of the facts of heredity for the benefit of the race."[62] In suggesting that genetics could serve the physician as a branch of "preventive medicine," these persons had eugenic motives in mind.

These individuals were not eugenicists of the old school; indeed, they belittled the goals and values of the earlier eugenicists. Snyder spent his college summers working at the Carnegie Institution's genetics laboratory at Cold Spring Harbor, which Davenport directed. He was grateful to Davenport for encouraging his interest in human genetics, but, as Snyder puts it, "I quickly became certain that the philosophy of the near-by Eugenics Record Office would require considerable improvement."[63] These new spokesmen expressed cautious views; they did not misrepresent the state of genetic science; they rejected earlier eugenicists' Social Darwinistic assumptions about man and society. Whereas former eugenicists had spoken of such vague and questionable "genetic conditions" as criminality, alcoholism, prostitution, and pauperism, these individuals were concerned with specific inherited medical diseases. Unlike earlier eugenicists, they urged voluntary compliance, not compulsion; segregation of defectives, not sterilization. Nonetheless, they also recognized that many diseases have hereditary backgrounds, and they felt that for eugenic reasons prospective parents afflicted with such conditions should have access to informed, sympathetic counseling when deciding whether or not to have children. They were arguing, in short, for the development of heredity clinics, and their pleas constituted the beginning not only of the instruction of genetics to medical students but also of today's genetic counseling services.

These pioneers did not originate the idea of genetic counseling. Though it was one of the less publicized aspects of the eugenics program, such

61. *Ibid.*, p. 158.
62. E. P. Lyon, "Heredity as a Subject in the Medical Curriculum," *Journal of the Association of American Medical Colleges*, 7(1932):299.
63. Laurence H. Snyder to author, December 3, 1970.

counseling was actually performed at the Eugenics Record Office and was a function that even the most orthodox eugenicist of old heartily approved. Snyder, Macklin, Allan, and others did recognize the importance of this part of the eugenic program, however, and they attempted to separate it from more pretentious eugenic suggestions. At an important symposium on genetic counseling in 1934, Sir Humphry Rolleston, president of the English Eugenics Society, stated:

> There is some confusion in the public mind about the meaning of the word eugenics; many still regard it as connoting such measures as the compulsory mating of selected individuals on the lines of the methods employed in the stockyard, or the compulsory sterilization of those somewhat vaguely labelled as unfit. To others, and among them members of the medical profession, the propaganda of eugenicists appear to have outrun the existing knowledge of the laws of human heredity. The principles of eugenics, however, can be defined in terms acceptable to most medical men who should then agree that the practice of what may be called negative eugenics [in the form of genetic counseling, the subject of the symposium] is the most effective, economical, and humane of the departments of preventive medicine.[64]

In 1948 the accumulated records of the Eugenics Record Office were transferred to the Dight Institute of the University of Minnesota, one of America's first agencies to offer genetic counseling services.[65] In England also a renovated Eugenics Education Society under the leadership of C. P. Blacker widely promoted genetic counseling. Today's heredity clinics, therefore, have descended directly from the early eugenics movement. Eugenic thought, in a precise, unpretentious form, has survived the original movement. Eugenics has divorced itself from Spencerian sociology and entered medicine.

In the 1950's further discoveries in human genetics strengthened the relationship between genetics and medicine. One important area of investigation consisted of work in biochemical and molecular genetics and in the study of hereditary diseases involving enzyme deficiencies. The theoretical understanding of the mechanism of gene action provided by molecular biologists impressed physicians, for it showed them that the science of genetics has physiological significance. The practical importance of bio-

---

64. Sir Humphry Rolleston, "Introduction," in C. P. Blacker, ed., *The Chances of Morbid Inheritance* (Baltimore: William Wood and Company, 1934), p. ix.

65. Lee R. Dice, "Heredity Clinics: Their Value for Public Service and for Research," *American Journal of Human Genetics*, 4(1952):9. The Dight Institute was organized in 1941. The first heredity clinic in the United States, other than the Eugenics Record Office, was the heredity clinic of the University of Michigan, established in 1940. (*Ibid.*, pp. 9–10.)

chemical genetics to medicine became apparent when Gerty T. Cori and Carl F. Cori demonstrated in 1952 the first specific enzyme defect in an inborn error of metabolism, the deficiency of glucose-7-phosphatase in Von Gierke's disease, one of the glycogen storage diseases. The following year George Jervis demonstrated that phenylketonuria (PKU) is caused by a deficiency of the enzyme phenylalanine hydroxylase, and since then medical scientists have discovered enzyme abnormalities in a multitude of "inborn errors." (At the time of this writing there are ninety-two diseases in which specific enzyme defects have been demonstrated.)[66] If diagnosed early enough, some of these diseases can be successfully treated. An appropriate diet, for example, apparently will enable a PKU baby to grow up without developing the mental deficiency normally associated with the disease. Such examples rendered absurd the notion that hereditary conditions are untreatable and illustrated the principle that genes determine the potential while environment determines the manifestations much more convincingly than did the earlier recognized genetic conditions like hemophilia or cleft palate.

A second important line of research involved studies of cytological and chromosomal genetics. In 1959 several major breakthroughs were achieved: C. E. Ford, P. A. Jacobs and colleagues discovered the role of the Y chromosome in sex determination in man; Peter Nowell and David Hungerford discovered the first specific chromosomal aberration associated with cancer in man; and Jerome Lejune discovered the first congenital malformation, Mongolian idiocy or "Down's syndrome," to be caused by a chromosomal abnormality. To pragmatic physicians, the idea that something visible in the cell, not just hypothetical "factors," caused a patient's condition was persuasive evidence for the importance of genetics to medicine.

Finally, the scope of human genetics was broadened in the 1950's to include the genetics of micro-organisms important to disease. Biologists in that decade began to show increasing interest in the topic of genetic resistance to chemotherapeutic agents among parasites. The whole subject received enormous attention in 1959 when T. Watanabe discovered the existence of resistance-transfer factors (RTF's) in certain strains of intestinal bacteria. The RTF is a type of episome (a particle of genetic material in bacteria which exists in the cytoplasm of the cell independent of the chromosome) which enables the microbe to resist the action of one or more drugs. These factors can be transferred from one bacterium to another in a process called "conjugation," the bacteria's equivalent of sexual reproduction. In this way drug immunity can be transferred to a

66. McKusick, "Human Genetics," pp. 8–11.

whole population of microbes. The importance of these findings to clinical situations was indisputable and immediately recognized.

With these developments the link between genetics and medicine became permanent, and medical genetics in the United States began its "takeoff." In the late 1950's medical genetics, as distinct from human genetics, became institutionalized.[67] The University of Washington School of Medicine formed a Division of Medical Genetics in 1956; the Johns Hopkins School of Medicine opened its Division of Medical Genetics in 1957; the University of Wisconsin School of Medicine established its Department of Medical Genetics in 1958; and others soon followed.[68] At the same time major medical foundations started to supply research and training grants to support work in genetics and human genetics. The National Foundation in 1958 began to sponsor research in congenital malformations, and since then it has established over one hundred birth defect centers which offer genetic counseling.[69] The National Heart Institute (today the National Heart and Lung Institute) and the National Institute of Neurological Diseases and Blindness (today the National Institute of Neurological Diseases and Stroke) in the late 1950's also started funding work in genetics; and the National Institute of General Medical Sciences and the National Institute of Child Health and Human Development, both established in 1962, began at once to support human genetics.[70] In the 1960's medical genetics continued to grow. Articles on genetic topics

67. Medical genetics is a discrete subspecialty of human genetics, even though the boundary between the two is arbitrary. A given department of either human or medical genetics is likely to contain investigators working on both clinical and non-clinical problems. The department of human genetics at the University of Michigan, for example, was organized in the 1940's as part of the Medical School and has always been involved with a very wide scope of activities.

68. The first department of medical genetics in America was actually established at the Bowman Gray School of Medicine at the time the school opened in 1941. Dean Carpenter of the developing new school had asked Snyder what he might do to make his institution unique and outstanding, and he had followed Snyder's suggestion of establishing a department of medical genetics. The department at Bowman Gray was therefore founded at least in part to help build the image of a new school; it did not indicate a "takeoff" in medical genetics. The institutionalization of medical genetics in the United States, as mentioned in the text, was to wait until the late 1950's. (Laurence H. Snyder to author, December 3, 1970.)

69. The National Foundation's support of research in birth defects may be followed in its *Annual Reports*.

70. Before becoming an institute, the National Institute of General Medical Sciences had divisional status; and in 1957, while still a division, it started a Training Grants Committee which supported work in genetics. All these institutes are parts of the National Institutes of Health. Information on the funding programs of the NIH is found in a brochure, *Basic Data Relating to the National Institutes of Health, 1970* (Washington, D. C.: Government Printing Office, June, 1970).

appeared in medical journals more and more frequently; between 1950 and 1970 the percentage of papers on such topics in the *Journal of Clinical Investigation* increased nearly ten-fold.[71] The percentage of physicians in the American Society of Human Genetics has approximately doubled since its beginning in 1948, and a few dozen dentists have also joined the Society.[72] (In 1956 the National Institute of Dental Research formed the first department of dental genetics in this country.[73]) Both a sign of medicine's increased interest in human genetics and a cause of the continued development of medical genetics is the Short Course in Medical Genetics, or the "Bar Harbor Course," held each summer in Bar Harbor, Maine. Organized and directed by members of the Jackson Laboratory and the Johns Hopkins University School of Medicine, the course is intended mainly for medical school faculty members. Since its inception in 1959, over 750 "students" have taken the course, including numerous senior faculty members, many department chairmen, and even a few deans.[74]

In the late 1950's medical genetics underwent a "takeoff" in other countries as well. Such a large number of medical doctors attended the Second International Congress of Human Genetics in Rome in 1961 that Luigi Gedda declared: "The Rome Congress, attended mostly by physicians and graced by the official presence of the authorities of Rome's Medical Faculty [which in 1961 established a chair in medical genetics], definitely sealed the link between Genetics and Medicine."[75]   The World Health Organization began to promote and disseminate knowledge of medical genetics; it started to sponsor training courses in the subject and symposia on specific genetic problems with medical applications. Mogens Hauge, a physician and editor of *Human Heredity* (an international journal published in Switzerland), says of his experiences as a director of four international training courses for medical school teachers from developing countries: "I have seen the very pronounced interest which medical people in these countries take in coming to know more about human genetics and in introducing the subject into their schools."[76] The first journal ex-

71. Personal copy of Barton Childs, "Genetics in Medicine," an address delivered to the Conference on Genetic Disease Control, Washington, D. C., December 2-5, 1970, Appendix.

72. Carl J. Witkop, Jr. to author, November 6, 1970.

73. Carl J. Witkop, Jr. to author, November 30, 1970.

74. Statistics obtained in conversation with Victor A. McKusick, November 3, 1970. Dr. McKusick, chairman of the Division of Medical Genetics of the Johns Hopkins University School of Medicine, helped create the course in 1959 and has been its co-director each year since.

75. Luigi Gedda, "Foreword," in *Proceedings of the Second International Congress of Human Genetics*, vol. 1, p. 12*.

76. Mogens Hauge to author, August 4, 1970.

clusively devoted to medical genetics, the *Journal of Medical Genetics*, was established in England in 1964.[77]

While human genetics in recent decades has contributed significantly to medical progress, the relationship has been reciprocal. In urging that genetics be added to the medical curriculum, Snyder, Macklin, and Allan recognized that physicians could contribute to human genetics as record gatherers. Snyder wrote in 1940:

> The study of human heredity has of course grown out of the experimental analysis of other organisms. It is assumed, on adequate grounds, that most of the great fundamental principles of heredity are now known. The work of the past forty years on a large variety of animals and plants has resulted in the establishment and understanding of these principles. It is now imperative to apply these principles to the various morphological, physiological, and pathological conditions in human beings, to test their validity in such conditions.[78]

In recent years medicine not only has been an area to confirm general genetic principles, as Snyder suggested, but in fact has made possible their elucidation. Interest in the disease sickle cell anemia led to A. C. Allison's demonstration in 1954 that infectious disease can influence the genetic constitution of man, and continued investigation of that disease resulted in Vernon Ingram's 1957 work which showed that the gene acts by determining the amino acid sequence of proteins—a study based on his comparison of sickle hemoglobin and normal hemoglobin A of man.

Today, medical genetics has progressed to a point where students in virtually every American medical school receive instruction in genetics, though not everywhere is the subject offered as a separate course. The prestige of human genetics or of genetics as a field of research at medical schools varies, being highest at those dozen or so major centers where formal departments or divisions of human genetics are established. Even at these places, it must be remembered that in terms of prestige human and clinical genetics must compete against areas in which discoveries can lead to procedures of immediate life-or-death importance in emergencies, such as X-rays or surgery. At the present time almost every medical student graduates with a knowledge of basic genetic principles and an appreciation of the role of heredity in disease, though few are then qualified to offer genetic counseling advice. Medical genetics has today reached the status of

77. *Acta Genetica et Statistica Medica*, founded by Gunnar Dahlberg in 1948 and re-named *Human Heredity* in 1969, has always aimed itself particularly at physicians, but its subject matter encompasses the entire field of human genetics, not just clinical genetics.
78. Snyder, *Medical Genetics*, p. 4.

a medical specialty and, like any medical specialty, requires post-graduate training to enter. This perhaps is how it should be, for in the application of genetics, more so than with most subjects, a little knowledge can be a dangerous thing. As long as medical genetics is pursued by the knowledgeable, its future seems secure.

4. Radiation and Human Genetics

While the intellectual reconstruction of human genetics was progressing, the United States dropped the atomic bomb on Hiroshima and Nagasaki. The advent of the atomic age did much to stimulate the further development of the science. Though workers in human genetics had already accomplished much in the way of laying a solid scientific groundwork in the subject, the atomic age gave these developments added impetus. Immediately after Hiroshima both scientists and laymen became greatly concerned over the potential genetic hazards of increased exposure to radiation. Certainly some individuals, most notably H. J. Muller, had worried about the genetic effects of radiation before the bomb, but the arrival of the atomic era gave the problem a pronounced immediacy. Public interest accordingly focused upon human genetics as a means of understanding and meeting the problem, and work in the field proceeded with a practical imperative.[79]

Prior to World War II most individuals assumed a cavalier attitude toward the use of radiation, even though its injurious somatic effects were almost immediately recognized.[80] Elihu Thomson in 1896, N. S. Scott in 1897, and E. A. Codman in 1902 were among those who quite early had pointed to the dangers of radiation and who had urged that great caution be employed in its use. With H. J. Muller's epoch announcement in 1927 of the artificial inducement of mutations in Drosophila by X-rays, the

79. Even today knowledge of man's response to radiation is very incomplete. A debate is still in progress regarding whether low levels of radiation will produce genetic damage in humans, and responsible scientists can be found on both sides of the issue. Enough information has been obtained, however, to show that many individuals at the end of World War II exaggerated the extent to which radiation is a genetic hazard to man. They made many claims that existing levels of fall-out might cause drastic genetic damage to human populations. Though their fear of radiation was later seen to be unwarranted, at the time it was so great that it led to the centering of interest on human genetics now to be discussed.

80. Material of this paragraph is obtained primarily from K. Z. Morgan, "History of Damage and Protection from Ionizing Radiation," in K. Z. Morgan and J. E. Turner, eds., *Principles of Radiation Protection* (New York: John Wiley & Sons, 1967); and also from Professor Donald Fleming, "Lectures in the History of Science in America," Harvard University.

menace of radiation should have been completely obvious.[81] Yet, early pleas for caution in the use of radiation were largely ignored. Not until 1916 did the Röntgen Society initiate the first organized efforts to promote methods of radiation protection, and its warnings about over-exposure to radiation were disregarded. (Later studies calculated that if the suggestions of the Röntgen Society had been followed, much of the death and suffering caused by overexposure to radiation during the next twenty years could have been averted. Only in very recent times have measures of radiation protection come to be required by law.) Numerous tragedies resulted from the careless use of radiation. By 1922 it had been estimated that over one hundred radiologists had died of occupationally produced cancer, and many later studies showed that radiologists have life expectancies shorter than those of other types of physicians. During World War I a group of women employed in the radium-dial painting industry ingested radium by virtue of their practice of tipping radium-coated paint-brushes with their lips and fifteen years later died early deaths from various types of cancer. As late as the 1920's reputable New York doctors used X-rays in cosmetic treatments to remove hairs from their lady patients, a practice the American Medical Association condemned only in 1929 despite earlier estimates that this practice had caused thousands of cases of burns and deaths.

Despite these accidents, there were compelling reasons why the public in this early period did not overly fear radiation. Since its discovery in 1895 radiation had found important medical applications, particularly to diagnosis and to the treatment of undesired growths. Journalists had widely publicized radiation as a miracle cure, as a powerful weapon to combat numerous maladies—including cancer. Moreover, since the body possesses no built-in sensory detection system against ionizing radiation, many of the side effects of radiation treatment frequently went unrecognized. Radiation effects often were not observed at the time of exposure; harmful consequences frequently were never attributed to the source. Even some of those who did worry about the somatic and genetic consequences of radiation were themselves careless when using it. Muller, of all people, in the late 1920's and early 1930's used to leave the lead box to turn the capsules containing flies while the radiation machine was running! He and his students suspected that radiation might have an effect on man, but they had not yet given serious thought to that possibility.[82] Small

81. Note that the importance of Muller's work was *immediately* recognized by his peers. In 1927, the year he made the discovery, he received for that work the AAAS Prize of $1000.
82. Clarence P. Oliver to author, August 4, 1970. As a graduate student Oliver worked in Muller's laboratory.

wonder, then, that others less knowledgeable than Muller gave the dangers of radiation little heed.[83]

With the first detonation of the atomic bomb this situation immediately and dramatically changed. In 1946 Muller received the Nobel Prize for his discovery that X-rays greatly increase the mutation rates of genes, and he declared in his address upon receiving the award:

It becomes an obligation for radiologists—though one far too little observed as yet in most countries—to insist that the simple precautions are taken which are necessary for shielding the gonads, whenever people are exposed to such radiation, either in industry or medical practice. And, with the coming increasing use of atomic energy, even for peace-time purposes, the problem will become very important of insuring that the human germ plasm—the all-important material of which we are the temporary custodians—is effectively protected from this additional and potent source of radiation.[84]

As radiation became a major controversy, public attention turned toward human genetics. The highly publicized studies of the somatic and genetic effects of the atomic bomb brought the discipline a large amount of notice.[85] So also did the reports of the National Academy's Committee on Biological Effects of Atomic Radiations and a series of widely followed Congressional hearings, particularly those held by the Holifield Joint Committee on Atomic Energy, in which geneticists played prominent roles. With the development of the hydrogen bomb and the spread of atomic know-how to other countries, concern over the genetic effects of radiation increased still further, and the public looked even more anxiously to human genetics to help explain the problem. Lionel Penrose wrote: "In recent years, moreover, there has been widespread speculation about the hereditary changes—that is, mutations—likely to be caused by the in-

83. L. J. Stadler, who co-discovered the mutagenic effect of radiation, was another researcher who quite early suspected that radiation might constitute a genetic danger to man. When performing experiments involving radiation emitters he was careful to take precautions for himself and for the people who worked with him. Nonetheless, he made no public warnings about the hazards of radiation. He was a much quieter man than Muller and was not given to speaking publicly. (Herschel L. Roman to author, January 11, 1971.)

84. Hermann J. Muller, "Production of Mutations. Nobel Lecture, December 12, 1946," in *Nobel Lectures, Physiology or Medicine, 1942–1962* (Amsterdam: Elsevier Publishing Co., 1964), p. 171.

85. See James V. Neel and W. J. Schull, eds., *The Effect of Exposure to the Atomic Bombs on Pregnancy Termination in Hiroshima and Nagasaki* (Washington, D. C.: National Academy of Sciences-National Research Council, 1956). This is the report of the Atomic Bomb Casualty Commission. See also Ashley W. Oughterson and Shield Warren, eds., *Medical Effects of the Atomic Bomb in Japan* (New York: McGraw-Hill, 1956). This volume represents the work of the Joint Commission for the Investigation of the Effects of the Atomic Bomb in Japan.

creased amount of ionizing radiation to which the human race may now be exposed in the atomic age just beginning. Information on this question is difficult to obtain and puzzling to evaluate except upon the basis of a sound knowledge of human genetics."[86] The continued peacetime development and use of atomic energy made the results of the First International Congress of Human Genetics of great topical interest. The United Nations requested to be informed of the results of the meeting, and the World Health Organization sent a group of its own experts to the congress to discuss and to evaluate its findings.[87] Russia's giant atomic bomb blast of 1961 occurred while the Second International Congress of Human Genetics was in session and brought that conference considerable publicity.

This increased public exposure worked to the advantage of human genetics. First and most obvious, the atomic age opened up new avenues of research in the subject; radiation genetics, mutagenesis, and the study of radiation-induced chromosomal aberrations became parts of its domain. Though the study of the genetic effects of radiation had been a fertile area of investigation since the 1920's, the advent of the atomic age significantly affected the field. In the late 1940's radiation genetics began to grow enormously in size and scope, and literature on the subject began to proliferate. After the war, radiation genetics also began to include the study of man as well as Drosophila and maize. At each of the three international congresses of human genetics, radiation genetics has been an important theme, particularly at the first congress where it was one of the central topics.[88] Much recent work in radiation genetics has continued to employ Drosophila or mouse as experimental subjects, but a considerable part of this research has been inspired by an awareness that humans too are vulnerable to radiation-induced genetic alterations, and much knowledge of mutation rates and mechanisms in man has been obtained from laboratory experiments with these lower organisms. In this instance the sphere of human genetics has come to extend beyond the customary limits of man as the experimental subject.

86. Lionel S. Penrose, *Outline of Human Genetics* (London: Heinemann, 1959), p. xi.

87. These facts are recorded in Julius Bomholt, "Opening Address," in *Proceedings of the First International Congress of Human Genetics*, pp. XI-XII.

88. At the first congress T. C. Carter went so far as to say, "Estimation of the dysgenic effect of a mutation rate increase requires detailed knowledge of the genetic mechanism underlying the illnesses which constitute the social load; obtaining this knowledge is the first task facing human geneticists." (T. C. Carter, "Radiation Genetics and Human Populations," in *Proceedings of the First International Congress of Human Genetics*, p. [47].)

In addition, the atomic age provided human genetics with important new sources of financial support. Even during the war a large project in radiation genetics was sponsored by the Manhattan Engineering Project. The major portion of that work was conducted at the University of Rochester, where investigators performed a range of studies of the pathological and genetic efforts of both acute and chronic irradiation.[89] The wartime Manhattan Project continued as the peacetime Atomic Energy Commission, and the AEC from its outset displayed a strong interest in population and radiation genetics, particularly in reference to man. In a booklet in 1949,[90] the AEC declared its commitment to support basic biological and medical research and outlined its entire program for medicine and biology. The booklet included a detailed listing of the AEC's major research centers; the AEC's unclassified contracts for biological, medical, and physical research; citations of volumes recording the Manhattan Project's wartime investigations in medicine and biology; and a list of the pre-and post-doctoral fellows supported by the AEC. (In 1949–50 the AEC provided a predoctoral fellowship to a young man at the University of Indiana who was soon to do his Nobel Prize winning work on unraveling the molecular structure of DNA—James D. Watson.[91]) Though individual examples are too numerous to supply, throughout the past two decades the AEC has continued to support basic research in genetics and human genetics. It has supplied fellowships to graduate students and postdoctoral fellows, research grants to investigators, and direct subsidies to university departments of human genetics; it also has established its own research centers like those at Oak Ridge and Argonne. Other organizations concerned with atomic energy have similarly promoted research in human genetics. The Subcommittee on Radiobiology of the Committee on Nuclear Science of the National Academy of Sciences–National Research Council, for example, has sponsored many research symposia on various aspects of radiobiology, beginning with the first symposium held at Oberlin College in 1950. The proceedings of many of these meetings later appeared in published form. The bomb made such an impression on the tax-paying public that it unhesitatingly allowed major increases in financial support to human genetics. Oak Ridge's one-million-dollar-a-year project studying the genetic effects of radiation on mice was easily justified; and popular books on the genetic effects of radiation, such as Bruce Wallace

89. This work was published in Henry Blair, ed., *Biological Effects of External Radiation* (New York: McGraw-Hill, 1954).
90. United States Atomic Energy Commission, *Atomic Energy and the Life Sciences* (Washington, D. C.: United States Government Printing Office, 1949).
91. *Ibid.*, p. 187.

and Theodosius Dobzhansky's *Radiation, Genes, and Man,* could plead without embarrassment for the support of future research in human genetics.[92]

The atomic age also helped attract new scientists to the field of human genetics. James V. Neel, who co-directed the Atomic Bomb Casualty Commission which studied the genetic effects of the atomic bomb on the population of Japan, was one who was so influenced. Neel received his Ph.D. in 1939 under Curt Stern at the University of Rochester, where he was trained as a Drosophila geneticist. As a graduate student he also began to develop an interest in human genetics, and over the next few years he decided to pursue the subject. In 1941 he entered medical school at Rochester with advanced student standing so he could be better equipped to handle the problems of human genetics. When his military number came up, he sought out the assignment with the ABCC; he considered that position the best opportunity to do human genetics that the United States military could offer someone with his background. He received the assignment, an event which started his own interest in mutagenesis and which provided genetics an early start at the ABCC.[93] The atomic age had a similar effect upon the career of William J. Schull, Neel's friend and colleague and the other co-director of the ABCC study. After training in human genetics under David Rife and Madge Macklin at Ohio State University in the period immediately following the war, he began working for the ABCC. His experience with that group strengthened his interest in mutagenesis and fortified his still stronger interest in human population genetics.[94] The ABCC project helped influence others who participated in it to choose careers in human genetics; Stanley W. Wright, a classmate of Neel at the University of Rochester School of Medicine and Dentistry, also became interested in genetics in 1950 while working on that project.[95] In subsequent years many young men have continued to enter human genetics because of a desire to study the genetic effects of radiation.

The atomic age also contributed to the campaign to add genetics to the medical school curriculum. Probably the most important example was the establishment of a medical genetics program in 1958 at the University of Wisconsin, which was a pioneer in the institutionalization of medical genetics in America. The major figure instituting the program was John Z. Bowers, now president of the Macy Foundation, who was dean of Wiscon-

92. See Bruce Wallace and Theodosius Dobzhansky, *Radiation, Genes, and Man* (New York: Holt, 1959), pp. 179–83.
93. James V. Neel to author, November 2, 1970.
94. William J. Schull to author, November 24, 1970.
95. Stanley W. Wright to author, December 3, 1970.

sin's medical school. Bowers' long-standing friendship with Joshua Leder-berg, who was then a professor of genetics at Wisconsin, was a main reason behind the initiation of the program. Lederberg stimulated Bowers to think seriously about the importance of developing a department of medi-cal genetics, and Bowers, recognizing Lederberg's greatness, desired to have him associated with the medical school. In addition, Bowers' experiences at the U. S. Atomic Energy Commission from 1947 to 1950 as Deputy Director of the Division of Biology and Medicine were a major factor in his developing the program. As Deputy Director he was involved in support of the Atomic Bomb Casualty Commission program at Hiroshima and Nagasaki and closely followed the genetics study led by Neel and Schull. He became quite "genetics conscious" and consequently was receptive to the idea of a medical genetics department when the proper circumstances arose later at Wisconsin.[96]

The atomic age also had a more subtle consequence for human genetics: it crystallized the problem of the "genetic load." Earlier geneticists, as noted in Chapter 3, had pointed out that medicine could save many of those afflicted with genetic defects, but a wide concern that the welfare state and modern medicine were drastically reducing the impact of natural selection did not develop until after Hiroshima. The term "genetic load" was originated by H. J. Muller, the leading publicist of the problem, in 1949.[97] Producing Muller's concern was his conviction that increases in background radiation were causing a sharp rise in the number of muta-tions. He repeatedly warned that this increased mutation rate, combined with the successful treatment of carriers of defective genes, might be pro-ducing a marked deterioration in the genetic quality of the human race. Hiroshima thus transformed an incipient controversy into a major public issue.[98]

Finally, the atomic age resulted in a display of social responsibility among human geneticists over the issue of atomic energy. As holders of the detailed knowledge of the biological effects of radiation, they felt obligated to publicize this knowledge in the hope that the major powers

96. John Z. Bowers to author, August 25, 1970.
97. H. J. Muller, "Our Load of Mutations," *American Journal of Human Genetics*, 2(1950):111–76. This paper was a longer version of his presidential address, "Our Mutations," which he delivered to the second annual meeting of the society in December, 1949.
98. Worry over the "genetic load" in turn gave impetus to the development of genetic counseling as a means to solve the dilemma. Lee R. Dice began his 1951 presidential address on heredity clinics to the American Society of Human Genetics by suggesting that the "genetic load" has produced a greater need for genetic coun-seling services. (Dice, "Heredity Clinics," p. 1.)

might use it to create sane nuclear policies. Resolutions on atomic weapons were passed by both the First and Second International Congresses of Human Genetics. These resolutions urged that the nations of the world construct agreements prohibiting the further development and use of nuclear weapons and that they conduct further research on the genetic effects of the peaceful use of atomic energy so that effective control measures might be formulated and instituted.[99]

It is not surprising that the development of atomic energy should have had these effects on human genetics. The initial post-war prosperity and sense of well-being were soon shattered by subsequent national and world events: the realization that wartime ally Russia is now a foe; the beginning of the Cold War; the fall of China; the Alger Hiss epsiode of 1949; the highly publicized espionage cases of the Rosenbergs and of Klaus Fuchs; the Korean War; and the shrill accusations of Senator Joe McCarthy. This general anxiety which plagued the American people was intensified by the dour realization that the atomic age with all its hazards was here permanently. Russia's development of the atomic bomb in 1949, the development of the hydrogen bomb in the 1950's, and a series of widely publicized accidents in which many individuals were exposed to fall-out radiation following nuclear test detonations all pointed to the imminency of the problem. A profound anxiety arose among all people concerning the influence of technology on the nature of any future global conflict, and the fall-out issue surpassed all other biological issues of the day (such as the fluoridation of water, non-radioactive air pollution, and the injurious effects of smoking) in its importance as a major factor in international relations.[100] It became quite natural to support research in human genetics as a means of giving these great anxieties a tangible focus and as a way to cope with the possible future consequences of nuclear technology. In a more positive and optimistic vein, research in human radiation genetics could also be justified as part of the program to develop atomic energy for peaceful purposes. Such a rationale was given by Lewis L. Strauss, Chairman of the United States Atomic Energy Commission, in the volume which recorded the Manhattan Project's wartime research on the genetic effects of radiation:

99. See *Proceedings of the First International Congress of Human Genetics*, p. (65); and *Proceedings of the Second International Congress of Human Genetics*, vol. 1, p. 34*.

100. The issue of fall-out comprised a major part of Adlai Stevenson's 1956 campaign for President. This made him the first Presidential candidate ever to make a scientific issue a main burden of his campaign.

As a result of conditions in the world, external to the United States, the requirements of national security have been paramount in our development of this industry [atomic energy] so far. Constant and increasing attention, however, has been given to the problems of economic nuclear power and to the medical and industrial applications of radioactive materials with a view toward "improving the public welfare, increasing the standard of living, strengthening free competition in private enterprise, and promoting world peace." To this end the Atomic Energy Commission has sought the most effective means to accelerate the practical exploitation of nuclear data to American science and industry.[101]

Though the atomic age stimulated the growth of human genetics, it provided an impetus to other fields as well. The Atomic Energy Commission recognized quite early that a study of the biological effects of radiation would not only establish safe levels of radiation exposure but would also yield discoveries of general importance. Henry A. Blair, who helped supervise the wartime work at the University of Rochester, wrote: "There seems to be no doubt, however, as is already evidenced in genetics, that studies of the effects of radiation will ultimately extend knowledge of biochemical processes far beyond the limited objectives of therapeutic radiology or the establishment of safe levels of human exposure."[102] Since the war the use of tracer methods employing radioactive isotopes has made possible many major discoveries in biology and chemistry. Though isotopes had been used experientially as early as the 1920's, they became available in large and inexpensive quantities only with the development of the atomic energy industry, which produced enormous numbers of them as by-products of the cyclotron.[103]

Thus, the advent of the atomic age gave great impetus to the development of human genetics in the United States. The discipline in one sense benefited from the fortuitous circumstance that Muller made his classic discovery of the mutagenic effect of radiation in the generation before the atomic bomb. Had this not been the case, then after Hiroshima and Nagasaki attention might have been paid solely to the determination of the somatic effects of radiation. No one in the bombs' aftermath might have thought to investigate the genetic consequences for the population of Japan. Human genetics thus profited from America's support of a program of balanced scientific research.

101. Lewis L. Strauss, "Foreword," in Blair, *Biological Effects*, p. v.
102. Henry Blair, "Volume Editor's Preface," *ibid.*, p. xiii.
103. The use of radioisotopes also stimulated the birth of new industries to produce equipment for the handling and assaying of isotopes.

9

Conclusion

The interaction between science and society is complex, often subtle and sometimes indirect. Scientific principles have been invoked in the formulation of national policy and the passage of federal laws. Genetic theories played such a role in the enactment of the statewide eugenic sterilization measures, the sterilization laws of Nazi Germany, and the Immigration Restriction Act of 1924. Passage of those laws required popular sentiment in their behalf, but the genetic arguments advanced by members of the eugenics movement helped organize and direct that sentiment. In return the political episodes mentioned above had repercussions for the science of genetics. Eugenicists' misuse of genetic theories spurred many geneticists, including some who once had been sympathetic to eugenics, to denounce the movement publicly. In addition, the excesses of eugenicists created an attitude of distrust toward the field of human genetics which for a while discouraged many biologists from pursuing the subject. Human genetics and eugenics were eventually resurrected with the coming of the atomic age, when great public interest in questions of human heredity and the "genetic load" was aroused.

It is not surprising that genetics has been so involved in twentieth-century American politics, for its intellectual content bears directly upon political matters in a way unlike that of any other science. The "nature-nurture" issue is fundamentally a biological problem, but its social and political significance is immense. A theory of the origin of the universe simply does not carry the same type of social import—for twentieth-century civilization, at least—as a theory of man's nature. By its very character genetic science is intimately related to society.[1]

1. I am distinguishing social issues from more general philosophical questions and suggesting that genetics has a unique relation only to the former.

⅄ As an instrument of social policy in the United States, genetics has been highly effective but not all-powerful. Many eugenicists used genetic arguments in urging selective immigration restriction before World War I, yet their pleas were heeded only in the changed social climate which followed the war. Though many geneticists (and anthropologists) renounced the eugenics movement in the 1920's, the movement survived until the 1930's when the social atmosphere created by the Depression and the rise of Hitler finally made many former eugenic sympathizers hostile to doctrines of racial superiority. It would seem from these events that if a scientific theory is to be used successfully to promote a social or political cause, the science involved cannot be divorced from the social and political sentiments of the day. Men are not blind slaves of passion, taking from science only to support preconceived opinions; but if a scientific theory is to influence public policy, it is most effective when operating within a social context already sympathetic with the goals of the theory's promulgators.

The effect of society upon genetics has been manifested in various ways. Emotional biases as well as social and political events have influenced the science. Early in the century the erroneous belief of many physicians that hereditary forces are omnipotent contributed to the medical profession's early disinterest in matters of inheritance. Human genetics suffered from its early involvement with the eugenics movement but benefited from the advent of the atomic age. Genetics has also been vulnerable to economic forces; after World War II much progress in the field was made possible by the increase in government science spending.

With scientific research now so costly and so dependent on government support, the greatest single "external" control on scientific investigation in the United States is economic. In the past, the American government generally has not used its economic power to direct science (the recent report of the House Subcommittee on Science, Research, and Development points out the absence of any clear national science policy), but it has the capability. Though the merits of a directed program of research may be debated, it appears that in the most comprehensive case such a program might be hazardous. If large sums of money were available, but only for investigation in defined areas, a grossly unbalanced research program would be created. Moreover, complex political questions would have to be met: who is to decide the direction of science, and at what cost may the political predetermination of scientific inquiry justifiably proceed?

The direction of scientific research is not determined by economic forces alone. Political pressure directly affects science by asking it to solve questions it otherwise would not have to answer or be able to answer. In addition, society's ethical values and needs seem implicitly to guide the

direction of science. Though science possesses a certain internal intellectual autonomy, society sets limits which determine the domain of that
autonomy. Biologists must conduct their experiments according to strict
rules concerning the sanctioned use of human subjects and humane treatment of laboratory animals. These boundaries must not be transgressed.
The direction of science thus seems to be determined partially by the role
that society expects and demands that science fulfill.

In any discussion of the application of scientific discovery and the
control of scientific research, certain moral and ethical questions arise. Are
there areas of knowledge which, because of their disquieting social implications, should not be investigated? To what extent is an individual scientist
entitled reasonably to withhold his knowledge from society on the
grounds of moral or value judgment? Does the scientist possess some absolute right to interpose *his* value system between the fruit of his work and
the undesirable application of his discoveries to offensive social objectives?
Has he the right of veto or the right to act as a concurrent majority in the
John C. Calhoun tradition, negating the will of the social majority? To
what extent may society *compel* a scientist to cooperate against his will in
the application of his skills to social goals he finds revolting, or at least
morally objectionable? Who possesses the obligation to bring a
professionally trained person to task whenever he brings discredit upon the
scientific community—even in the furtherance of a socially popular cause?
With whom is to reside the ultimate authority and responsibility for the
social applications of science, and what shall be their criteria? The crux of
these questions seems to be the difficulty of defining a universal code of
scientific conduct acceptable even to members of the scientific community, not to mention politicians who may seek to control them.

What will be the future of eugenic applications in the United States? A
survey of contemporary American society offers no certain answer, only
ambiguous and contradictory signs. Contemporary medical research is con-
centrating more and more earnestly on controlling hereditary conditions,
having developed techniques and procedures which make possible the *in
utero* detection of fetuses afflicted with certain "inborn errors." At the
same time, however, medical interest has not diminished in the conquest
of disease by conventional environmental methods of surgery, diet, and
medication—an approach which if completely successful theoretically
would eliminate the need for any type of eugenic elimination of the particular deleterious genes.[2] As mentioned earlier in particular reference to

2. The author recalls a recent radio advertisement requesting contributions to
cancer research. Asserting that " 'Science' has found evidence that viruses cause
cancer," the ad suggested that the disease might be controllable since the culprit
appears to be environmental. It would seem that a fear of genetic causation is still a

genetic engineering, some current problems of human genetics are possibly in danger of being approached too objectively; yet the furor now raging over the suggestions of Stanford physicist William Shockley and Berkeley psychologist Arthur Jensen that blacks are intellectually inferior to whites indicates that other problems of human genetics are still laden with emotion.[3] Of course, there is no reason why eugenic and environmental approaches cannot be pursued simultaneously, but so far there is no concurrence regarding their relative desirability or potential effectiveness. Moreover, at a time when American society must determine how to permit individual expression without inviting lawlessness or civil disobedience and how to control crime and violence without instigating repression, the ancient problem of defining the responsibility of the individual to the group and of the present generation to posterity is as unresolved as ever; on no other issue is agreement so fundamental a prerequisite to the enactment of wide-scale eugenic measures.

The eugenics question aside, many other biological matters are currently political problems as well. The 1970's opened with marijuana, narcotics, the pill, the psychological effects of pornography, and ecology among the major political issues of the day. In discussion of these issues it is apparent that the same tendency to fit facts to policy rather than to build policy upon facts—so prominent in the debates over immigration restriction—still exists. The recent testimony of a host of scientific and medical experts that the harmful effects of marijuana have been greatly exaggerated made little noticeable impact upon congressmen. Conviction (at the time of this writing) remains a felony, and legal technicalities have made research into the drug's properties exceedingly difficult to carry out.[4] The conclusions of President Nixon's Commissions on Pornography

---

strong feature of American society and that an emphasis upon environmental etiology is still very useful when appealing to the public for the support of research.

3. Shockley, who in 1956 received the Nobel Prize in physics for discovering the transistor, has insisted for years that the average IQ of blacks is significantly less than that of whites. He has repeatedly urged the National Academy of Sciences to sponsor a detailed investigation of the question, but the academy has not yet done so. Jensen performed a study ("How Much Can We Boost I.Q. and Scholastic Achievement?" *Harvard Educational Review*, 39[1969]:1) in which he tested the IQ's of white and black children in each of several social-economic classes and found that white children on the average scored a standard deviation higher than black children of the same economic background. Since its publication this study has been attacked bitterly by liberal educators, sociologists, and psychologists. Regardless of whether the ideas of Shockley and Jensen have merit, the furor they created illustrates how taboo the question of racial differences has become as a subject for scientific pursuit since the time of Hitler. Some individuals have even suggested that the whole topic is better off not pursued at all.

4. I am not arguing that marijuana is harmless and should be legalized, nor am I suggesting that its biological effects are well understood. I am merely protesting the

(and on Campus Violence) were denounced by many, including the President himself, before the studies were officially released. Without having read the reports, numerous citizens and politicians, emotionally committed to conflicting views, challenged the commissions' "competence" and "authority." Today as in 1924, scientific argument cannot overcome irrational sentiment against a position, though it can be used effectively when scientific fact and sentiment happen to coincide. Perhaps it is not surprising that this is so, for the tendency to fit facts to policy is undoubtedly traceable to human nature—which, it would appear from the record afforded by history, has not changed in substance and which rises to throw askew the best-laid plans of politicians, generals, and yes, scientists too!

During the present controversy over applications of genetics, many geneticists are once again meeting their social responsibility by helping to guide public discussion of the issues. Though such efforts are needed, it must be realized that the exercise of social responsibility also involves certain dangers. Scientists may not always be able to safeguard themselves by distinguishing between their roles as *scientists* and *citizens*. A public accustomed to respect the authority of scientists may find it difficult to realize that some of their occasional remarks are imprecise and nonscientific. In important, emotionally laden issues a bewildered and anxious citizenry, noting that scientists in possession of the same facts hold contradictory opinions, may feel that science has somehow failed. In addition, some scientists may capitalize on the public's regard for them as experts to speak on issues outside their areas of authority, or they might inadvertently pass off speculation as fact. Though social responsibility is generally considered desirable, it would seem that it also carries the danger of being abused, and if this happens science may thereby incur some of the mistrust that traditionally belongs to politics.

Some feel that this is already happening today. There is a growing disillusionment with science among the young—a decreased enrollment in university science courses, renewed interest among youth in astrology, mysticism, and the occult. Such a revolt against science does not necessarily have to occur. At the heart of the problem lies not the failure of science but this century's unrealistic faith that science is without limitations. With such high expectations the disillusionment is correspondingly greater when science does not perform as anticipated. The solution, I think, lies in a more thorough education of the public on the true nature of science—on its limitations as well as its capabilities, on the degree to

---

justification of current prohibitions on marijuana for the *wrong* reasons, namely, the continued reference to putative biological effects of the drug which investigation has already shown it does not produce, such as the frequently made claim that repeated marijuana usage leads to heroin addiction.

which it may *reasonably* be expected to contribute to the solution of social problems, on the important distinction between fact and interpretation or speculation. The public must be taught to respect the scientific method and scientific fact without being duped into believing that they are omnipotent. With such an approach, it may be expected that science in America will continue to occupy a position of esteem.

Bibliographical Note

The footnotes provide a guide to the sources consulted in writing this book. Here I shall outline my approach and indicate the secondary works I found especially useful.

For understanding geneticists' attitudes toward the eugenics movement, the collections of the American Philosophical Society Library were indispensable. The library contains the correspondence and memoirs of several important geneticists, including Albert F. Blakeslee, William E. Castle, Charles B. Davenport, L. C. Dunn, Herbert S. Jennings, and T. H. Morgan; it also houses the University of California Genetics Department Papers. The Davenport and Jennings collections were particularly important for the years prior to 1930; the Dunn Papers, for the decade after 1930. Since I completed the book the library has expanded its genetics collections. The Dunn correspondence has been increased approximately three-fold, and papers of M. Demerec and H. J. Muller have been added.

The Correspondence of the House Committee on Immigration and Naturalization, located in the National Archives in Washington, D. C., was invaluable for discerning the influence of eugenic thought upon Albert Johnson and the diffusion of the biological argument for selective immigration restriction to the general public. Equivalent correspondence of the Senate Committee on Immigration was not available. Unfortunately, Johnson burned his personal papers. The Edward A. Ross Papers, at the State Historical Society of Wisconsin in Madison, and the files of the Immigration Restriction League, located in Harvard's Houghton Library, were moderately helpful for detecting the prejudices and viewpoints of some of the extreme restrictionists.

Toward the end of my research I carried on correspondence and conducted interviews with many of those who participated in the events discussed in the book. At this stage of the project I had acquired sufficient background to query my informants on specific matters but was not yet committed to particular ideas or interpretations. With one exception, all interviews lasted at least two hours; two were conducted over a period of several days. These activities proved to be extraordinarily helpful for confirming hypotheses, obtaining new leads, and acquiring illustrative anecdotes. Individuals I consulted are listed in the Preface.

The past decade has witnessed an awakening of historical interest in genetics. The reader may now choose from three histories of the science: Elof A. Carlson, *The Gene; A Critical History* (Philadelphia: W. B. Saunders Co., 1966); L. C. Dunn, *A Short History of Genetics* (New York: McGraw-Hill Co., 1965); and A. H. Sturtevant, *A History of Genetics* (New York: Harper and Row, 1965). Dunn's work was particularly helpful to this project, containing the most complete account of the development of human and population genetics. William B. Provine recently published *The Origins of Theoretical Population Genetics* (Chicago: University of Chicago Press, 1971) which chronicles the development of the subject from the time of Darwin through the classical era of the early 1930's. Much valuable historical information is contained in R. A. Brink, ed., *Heritage from Mendel* (Madison: The University of Wisconsin Press, 1967); L. C. Dunn, ed., *Genetics in the 20th Century* (New York: Macmillan Co., 1951); and the "Commemoration of the Publication of Gregor Mendel's Pioneer Experiments in Genetics," *Proceedings of the American Philosophical Society*, 109(1965):189–248. Though a book-length monograph on the history of human genetics has yet to appear, perceptive articles on the topic have been written by L. C. Dunn, "Cross Currents in the History of Human Genetics," *American Journal of Human Genetics*, 14(1962):1–13; Lionel Penrose, "Presidential Address—The Influence of the English Tradition in Human Genetics," *Proceedings of the Third International Congress of Human Genetics* (Baltimore: The Johns Hopkins Press, 1967); and Laurence H. Snyder, "Old and New Pathways in Human Genetics," *American Journal of Human Genetics*, 3(1951):1–16.

Much has been written about topics in American social and intellectual history relating to the subjects of this book. Two histories of the American eugenics movement are available: Mark H. Haller, *Eugenics: Hereditarian Attitudes in American Thought* (New Brunswick, N. J.: Rutgers University Press, 1963); and Donald K. Pickens, *Eugenics and the Progressives* (Nashville: Vanderbilt University Press, 1968). Despite its inattention to the naturalistic origins of the movement, Haller's lucid book is by far the more useful. The events leading up to the Immigration Restriction Act of 1924 are traced carefully by John Higham in *Strangers in the Land; Patterns of American Nativism 1860–1925* (New Brunswick, N. J.: Rutgers University

Press, 1955) and by Barbara Solomon in *Ancestors and Immigrants; A Changing New England Tradition* (Cambridge: Harvard University Press, 1956). An excellent discussion of the Johnson Act is found also in the first chapter of Robert A. Divine, *American Immigration Policy, 1924-1952* (New Haven: Yale University Press, 1957). Informative treatments of the history of racial thought are contained in Thomas F. Gossett, *Race: The History of an Idea in America* (Dallas: Southern Methodist University Press, 1963); John S. Haller, Jr., *Outcasts from Evolution: Scientific Attitudes of Racial Inferiority, 1859-1900* (Urbana, Ill.: University of Illinois Press, 1971); Oscar Handlin, *Race and Nationality in American Life* (Boston: Little, Brown and Co., 1957); and William Stanton, *The Leopard's Spots* (Chicago: University of Chicago Press, 1960). Other useful background sources include Oscar Handlin, *The Uprooted* (New York: Grosset and Dunlap, 1951); Richard Hofstadter, *Social Darwinism in American Thought*, rev. ed., (Boston: Beacon Press, 1955); Richard Hofstadter, *The Age of Reform from Bryan to F. D. R.* (New York: Alfred Knopf, 1955); Stow Persons, *American Minds: A History of Ideas* (New York: Henry Holt, 1958); and C. Vann Woodward, *The Strange Career of Jim Crow*, 2nd ed. (New York: Oxford University Press, 1966).

Index

of inheritance, 60–61, 80; as eugeni-
cist, 9, 20, 28, 34, 35, 36, 37, 42, 53n,
68n; *Heredity in Relation to Eugenics*,
50–51, 56–57, *How to Make a Eu-
genical Family Study*, 62; as human
geneticist, 48–49, 50, 51, 55, 57, 62,
70, 148, 155
Davis, James J., 104
Davison, Charles Stewart, 31, 96
Debs, Eugene, 98
Deutsche Gesellschaft für Rassen-
hygiene, 113–14
Diabetes mellitus, 68
Dice, Lee R., 199n
Dickstein, Samuel, 106
Differential birth rate, 35–37
Dight, Charles F., 18, 136
Dight Institute for the Promotion of Hu-
man Genetics, 136, 188
Dillingham, William, 96, 97
Dillingham Commission, 25, 97
Discontinuous traits, definition of, 45
Disharmonious crossings, theory of, 101,
102, 139
Dobzhansky, Theodosius, *Radiation,
Genes, and Man*, 198
Down's syndrome, 189
Dugdale, Robert, 36n
Dunn, L. C., 118, 126n, 136, 151, 181;
repudiates eugenics movement,
127–30

East, Edward M., 34, 80, 82, 121, 126n,
148, 151; and "biological sociology,"
38, 159; criticizes eugenics movement,
124; develops multiple-gene theory,
76–77; *Mankind at the Crossroads*,
124; supports eugenics movement, 37,
38, 40, 42, 43
Eaton, G. D., 82n
Emerson, Rollins A., 76–77, 80, 129
Environment: belief in predominance of,
5n, 127; recognition of interaction of
heredity and, 75–76, 80, 81, 102,
126–27
Essay on the Inequality of Races (Count
Arthur de Gobineau), 21
Eugenical News, 30n, 117, 177
*Eugenical Sterilization in the United
States* (Harry H. Laughlin), 92–93

Eugenics: definition of, 2; negative, 2,
7–8, 23, 46; positive, 2, 8, 46. *See also*
Eugenics movement
Eugenics Committee of the United
States of America, 89, 108
Eugenics Education Society, 137, 141,
156, 188; feud with Eugenics Laboratory, 54–55, 157
Eugenics Laboratory, 49, 50, 54–55,
157
Eugenics movement, 70–71, 84–85; attitudes of geneticists toward, 34–43,
79–83, 121–30, 131–34; class consciousness of, 20; in England, 156–57;
espouses view of Nordic superiority,
21–23; in Nazi Germany, 113–19,
127–28; origins of, 7, 9–14; platform
of, 7–9, 23, 53n, 81n, 90; racism of,
25–33, 84, 87–88; relation to state of
scientific knowledge of the day,
38–40, 75–79, 125–27; as a religion,
17–19, 38, 163; reorientation of philosophy of, in 1930's, 174–78; similarities between progressive movement
and, 15–19; static qualities of, 8–9,
15, 19–20; supports Nazi eugenic
measures, 117–19, 121, 128, 132. *See
also* Eugenics; Immigration Restriction
Act of 1924, influence of eugenics
movement on
Eugenics Quarterly, 177, 178
Eugenics Record Office, 7, 34, 43, 49n,
70, 169, 188; *Bulletins*, 50; criticism
of work of, 61, 79–80; *Memoirs*, 50;
promotes early work in human genetics, 48–49; sponsors uncritical research, 57, 58–59, 78
Eugenics Review, 178
Eugenic Sterilization Law, Nazi Germany, 31, 87, 116–17, 127–28
"Europe as an Emigrant-Exporting Continent" (Harry H. Laughlin), 101
Euthanasia law, Nazi Germany, 117
Evolution and Genetics (T. H. Morgan),
124
Evolution, Genetics, and Eugenics
(Horatio H. Newman), 51

Fairchild, David, 49n
Fairchild, Henry Pratt, 31, 108

THE JOHNS HOPKINS UNIVERSITY PRESS

This book was composed in Press Roman text with Avande Guarde
display by Jones Composition Company, Inc. from a design by
Laurie Jewell. It was printed on 60-lb. Sebago Regular stock
by Universal Lithographers, Inc. and bound in Holliston Payko
by L. H. Jenkins, Inc.

Library of Congress Cataloging in Publication Data

Ludmerer, Kenneth M
    Genetics and American society.

    Bibliography: p.
    1. Eugenics. 2. Human genetics. 3. United States—Social conditions.
I. Title.

HQ752.L77   301.24′3   72-4227
ISBN 0-8018-1357-3

DATE DUE